Self-Assessment Color Review

Adult Emergency Medicine

John F O'Brien MD

Associate Program Director/Emergency Medicine Residency
Orlando Regional Medical Center
Orlando, Florida, USA

Clinical Associate Professor of Emergency Medicine
University of Central Florida College of Medicine
Orlando, Florida, USA

Associate Professor of Emergency Medicine
Faculty of Emergency Medicine
University of Florida College of Medicine
Gainesville, Florida, USA

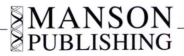

MANSON
PUBLISHING

Acknowledgements

I would like to thank several people who were instrumental in helping create this textbook. Many of my colleagues in Orlando helped with finding interesting cases, particularly Dr. Mark Clark. Several emergency medicine residents served as primary reviewers for much of the material in this endeavor, particularly Dr. Clifford Denney. My son, Nathan O'Brien, who recently completed his medical school training at Vanderbilt University and has begun his post-graduate training in emergency medicine, was perhaps the most detailed reviewer of all. The formal reviewers, Dr. John Younger and Dr. Peter Thomas, added many specific suggestions for improving the case discussions. Peter Beynon was a great help in word crafting the discussions to make them more interesting and succinct. Paul Bennett was instrumental in formatting the cases into an attractive casebook. My commissioning editor at Manson Publishing, Jill Northcott, was ever supportive in helping me accomplish this complicated task. Last, but most importantly, I wish to thank my wonderful wife Rhonda, who served as primary typist, organizer, and encourager. Without her tremendous help it is unlikely this would have ever been completed.

Copyright © 2013 Manson Publishing Ltd
ISBN: 978-1-84076-178-8

A CIP catalogue record for this book is available from the British Library.

For full details of all Manson Publishing Ltd titles please write to:
Manson Publishing Ltd, 73 Corringham Road, London NW11 7DL, UK.
Tel: +44(0)20 8905 5150
Fax: +44(0)20 8201 9233
Email: manson@mansonpublishing.com
Website: www.mansonpublishing.com

Commissioning editor: Jill Northcott
Project manager: Paul Bennett
Copy editor: Peter Beynon
Design and layout: Cathy Martin
Colour reproduction: Tenon & Polert Colour Scanning Ltd, Hong Kong
Printed by: New Era Printing Company Ltd, Hong Kong

Preface

The provision of competent emergency medical care is frequently both challenging and exhilarating. An ever-expanding knowledge base is necessary, coupled with clinical judgement and the ability to process often quite complex information. Much can be gained from experience in the emergency medicine clinical arena, and this self-assessment book attempts to assist in that endeavor through a case-based approach. Using a series of common as well as more unusual presentations, this text attempts to inform and refresh the reader across the entire spectrum of adult emergency medicine. Although pediatrics is not covered in these pages, a similar case book specific to children is available through this publisher. Medical trainees and qualified practitioners working not only in general emergency medicine, but also in primary care and other specialties, may use these cases to test and refine their abilities to care for a wide variety of patients.

This book employs questions to stimulate the reader to think about the evaluation and management of each patient, using a combination of photographs, radiographs, electrocardiograms, and other data. Discussions ensue, which should highlight various aspects of the case including differential diagnoses, management issues, and subtle insights to provide optimal care and prevent complications. Please enjoy the ride as you assimilate much of what is necessary to practice the art of emergency medicine.

Note that regional variations in the provision of emergency care exist. The reader should feel free to add to the learning experience by exploring the references attached to each case. In addition, specific practice guidelines should be sought from reliable local resources and societies. Clearly, a variety of management techniques can be thoughtfully applied to many clinical situations, and this book can only provide some evidence-based approaches.

John O'Brien

Classification of cases

Cardiology
1, 16, 45, 57, 73, 75, 91, 94, 102, 108, 112, 114, 120, 128, 131, 146, 147, 153, 157, 163, 165, 167, 176, 178, 182, 191, 197, 203, 207, 209, 217, 220, 225, 227, 232, 239, 245

Dermatology
18, 19, 24, 32, 38, 72, 76, 103, 110, 121, 127, 145, 162, 175, 181, 183, 184, 199, 208, 229, 233, 237, 242

Gastroenterology
5, 27, 35, 50, 62, 64, 74, 83, 100, 104, 115, 125, 139, 143, 151, 170, 173, 179, 195, 215, 246

Genitourinary
17, 42, 43, 47, 51, 52, 54, 71, 99, 118, 150, 161, 168, 211, 219, 231

Infectious disease
6, 11, 21, 25, 49, 68, 70, 82, 93, 101, 113, 119, 123, 124, 130, 132, 133, 152, 177, 223, 226, 250

Miscellaneous
12, 37, 41, 58, 59, 86, 87, 105, 111, 116, 141, 146, 159, 169, 189, 193, 198, 210, 221, 224, 249

Abbreviations

ABC	airway, breathing, and circulation
AIDS	acquired immunodeficiency syndrome
beta-hCG	beta human chorionic gonadotropin
BP	blood pressure
bpm	beats per minute
CBC	complete blood count
CNS	central nervous system
COPD	chronic obstructive pulmonary disease
CPR	cardiopulmonary resuscitation
CSF	cerebrospinal fluid
CT	computerized tomography
DBP	diastolic blood pressure
ECG	electrocardiogram
ELISA	enzyme-linked immunosorbent assay
FAST	focused assessment by sonography in trauma
GABA	gamma-aminobutyric acid
HAART	highly active anti-retroviral therapy
HIV	human immunodeficiency virus
INR	international normalized ratio
IV	intravenous/intravenously
LAD	left anterior descending (artery)
MRA	magnetic resonance angiography
MRI	magnetic resonance imaging
NSAID	nonsteroidal anti-inflammatory drug
NSR	normal sinus rhythm
P	pulse
P_{ox}	pulse oximetry
PCR	polymerase chain reaction
RBCs	red blood cells
RNA	ribonucleic acid
RR	respiratory rate
SAH	subarachnoid hemorrhage
SBP	systolic blood pressure
STEMI	ST segment elevation myocardial infarction
T	temperature
WBCs	white blood cells

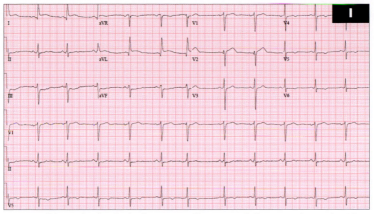

1 A 49-year-old male had diabetes mellitus and known hyperlipidemia. He presented with 2 hours of severe precordial chest pain, shortness of breath, and nausea. He appeared ill and was very diaphoretic.
i. What does this ECG suggest (1)?
ii. What are indications for reperfusion therapy?

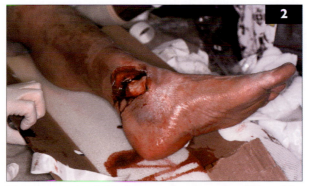

2 A 34-year-old male sustained this injury when he twisted his ankle while running (2).
i. What is the diagnosis?
ii. What associated complications are likely, and how should they be managed?

1 i. The ECG demonstrates normal sinus rhythm at about 70 bpm (premature atrial contraction in sixth beat). ST segments are elevated over 1 mm in lateral leads (I and aVL), with slight reciprocal ST depression in inferior leads III and aVF. T waves are inverted in leads V_4 to V_6. This is consistent with acute lateral wall myocardial infarction. Cardiac catheterization revealed acute LAD coronary artery occlusion.

ii. Rapid and aggressive management of acute myocardial infarction greatly reduces morbidity and mortality. New ST elevation of 1 mm or more in contiguous associated leads, in the setting of chest pain or anginal equivalents of recent onset (usually <6 hours from symptom onset, but even longer if stuttering course or ongoing ischemia), mandates reperfusion therapy. Associated leads are as follows: inferior leads: II, III, and aVF; lateral leads: I, aVL, V_5, and V_6; anterior leads: V_1 to V_4; posterior leads: V_7 to V_9; right ventricular leads: right-sided V_1 to V_6 (particularly right V_4). ECG changes for posterior wall myocardial infarction are seen indirectly in anterior precordial leads, with tall R waves in V_1 to V_3 with ST segment depression and upright T waves. New onset of left bundle branch block with suspected ongoing ischemia is also an indication for reperfusion therapy. Serial ECGs, and comparison to previous ones, is often helpful in borderline cases.

2 i. This is an open medial ankle injury, usually due to an eversion and external rotation mechanism. Associated deltoid ligament injury or medial malleolus avulsion is likely, and a spiral distal fibular fracture is usually present. Rarely, deltoid ligament or medial malleolus injuries are associated with a tear in the tibiofibular syndesmosis, often with a proximal fibular fracture. This is termed a Maisonneuve fracture and may lead to chronic ankle instability if not recognized and managed correctly. Occasionally, an open ankle can occur without fracture, particularly with penetrating trauma. Careful neurovascular examination is important. Simple radiographs are usually adequate to assess for fracture, with CT reserved for complex fractures.

ii. Liberal analgesia is indicated. Neurovascular status may be compromised by dislocation, in which case prompt reduction is indicated. Open fractures should be covered by wet sterile dressings. Broad-spectrum antibiotics and tetanus prophylaxis are indicated. Early orthopedic consultation is important since joint irrigation, exploration, and surgical repair are necessary.

3 A 32-year-old male presented 30 minutes after being an unrestrained passenger in a motor vehicle collision. He was talking, but a bit combative. BP was 80/54 mmHg (10.7/7.2 kPa) and P 156 bpm. He had clear lungs, a stable pelvis, no extremity injuries, and no evidence of significant external bleeding. He had moderate left upper quadrant pain.
i. What is the appropriate evaluation and management of this patient?
ii. Discuss some of the controversies in management?

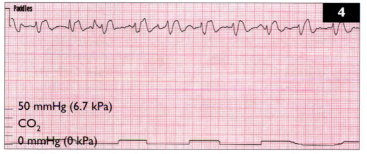

4 A 72-year-old female was intubated after cardiac arrest and had not recovered a pulse despite aggressive attempts at CPR.
i. What does her respiratory CO_2 waveform capnogram tell you (4)?
ii. Should CPR be continued?

3 i. Because of probable hemorrhagic shock, evaluation and management must be concomitant and expeditious. The patient appears to have a stable airway. IV access with two large caliber catheters should be obtained and crystalloid infused rapidly to improve perfusion. Laboratory tests include CBC along with type and cross-matching for packed RBCs. Chest and pelvis radiographs should be obtained. Ultrasound FAST techniques should look at the heart, hepatorenal, splenorenal, and bladder spaces to screen for intra-abdominal trauma. CT of the abdomen and pelvis is an alternative evaluation technique, but may cause dangerous delay if hemodynamic instability exists. Peritoneal lavage to evaluate for significant intra-abdominal bleeding has largely been supplanted by the above methods. Immediate surgical consultation is indicated. Decisions for operative intervention are often made clinically if evidence of significant intra-abdominal injury and/or hemodynamic instability exists. Packed RBCs should be infused if hypoperfusion persists after about 2 liters of crystalloid.

ii. Submaximal volume resuscitation to avoid increased bleeding may improve survival if rapid surgical intervention, with minimal IV fluids, is done quickly to repair bleeding intra-abdominal organs. Selective arterial embolization for bleeding hepatic and/or splenic injuries is used in some clinical settings. Nonoperative management of splenic or hepatic injuries is frequent when hemodynamic stabilization can be accomplished. However, fear of unrecognized associated intra-abdominal injuries and resultant complications makes nonoperative management controversial.

4 i. The monitor strip reveals an irregular wide-complex rhythm, which in this setting represents pulseless electrical activity. The capnographic waveform demonstrates an appropriate but small rise to about 8 mmHg (1.1 kPa) in CO_2 with exhalation, with return to zero during inhalation. This confirms appropriate endotracheal tube placement in the airway. However, the low expiratory CO_2 level in this setting suggests that minimal blood is being delivered to the lungs for ventilatory exchange. This confirms severe hypoperfusion to the brain, heart, and other organs as well, suggesting that CPR is inadequate. Sudden improvement in expiratory CO_2 levels with CPR suggests improved perfusion, but elevations may also occur with sodium bicarbonate administration, which can cause confusion if not understood.

ii. Attempts to improve CPR by more aggressive chest compression or other techniques should be considered. If expiratory CO_2 remains <10 mmHg (1.3 kPa) for more than a few minutes, continued efforts are likely to be futile.

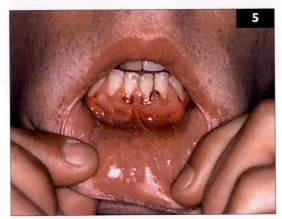

5 This 20-year-old male presented with a painful mouth, along with frequent bleeding from his gums over the past few days (5).
i. What is this problem, and what are the predisposing factors?
ii. How should it be treated?

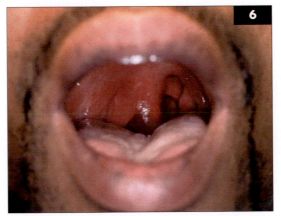

6 This 25-year-old patient had several days of severe sore throat with fever, diffuse myalgias, and increased fatigue (6). His streptococcal throat screen was negative.
i. What are the diagnostic considerations here?
ii. Is any therapy likely to help?

5 i. Acute necrotizing ulcerative gingivostomatitis (ANUG), also known as Vincent's angina or trench mouth. It was prevalent among soldiers stuck in the trenches during World War I. ANUG is a progressive, painful anterior mouth infection with swelling, ulceration, and gum necrosis. It may progress to involve the entire mouth and throat as well as cause dental loss. ANUG is typically caused by overgrowth of normal oral bacteria, including *Bacteroides*, *Fusobacterium*, and other anaerobic species. Factors such as poor oral hygiene, inadequate nutrition, stress, and other infections predispose to trench mouth. It has become increasingly common with AIDS. The patient presents with painful, swollen gums along with bad breath and foul taste. The gums are often hyperemic, with a gray film and ulcers between the teeth, and bleed with any irritation.
ii. Treatment begins with improved oral hygiene, using dilute hydrogen peroxide or saltwater rinses. Penicillin remains the antibiotic therapy of choice, although metronidazole is also used. Smoking cessation, proper nutrition, and improved dental care help with prevention. HIV testing may be indicated.

6 i. This is acute pharyngitis, usually due to various viral infections (adenovirus most commonly, but Epstein–Barr and HIV also important). Bacterial causes are mostly streptococcal, but *Corynebacterium diphtheriae*, *Neisseria gonorrheae*, *Chlamydia*, and *Mycoplasma* are other considerations. Recently, overgrowth of *Fusobacterium necrophorum*, a normal oral flora, has been implicated in formation of peritonsillar abscesses and/or Lemierre's syndrome (infectious thrombophlebitis of the internal jugular vein). *Candida albicans* and chemical irritants are other common etiologies. Throat pain, fever, difficulty swallowing, and headache are frequent with acute pharyngitis, along with various rashes and lymphadenopathy. Various antigen assays for *Streptococcus* may be useful, but false negatives related mainly to collection techniques and false positives due to chronic carrier state may occur. The global burden of rheumatic heart disease complicating streptococcal disease is found disproportionally in developing countries. Testing for infectious mononucleosis by a heterophile antibody test may be negative early, as sensitivity peaks at 2–6 weeks. CBC may show a suggestive increase in total lymphocytes to >60%, with atypical lymphocytes >10%. Primary HIV infection may cause a mononucleosis-like illness and should be considered in at-risk patients, with quantitative HIV-1 RNA viral load by PCR positive as early as 11 days after infection.
ii. Paracetamol and/or NSAIDs may provide effective pain relief. Penicillin remains the antibiotic of choice for streptococcal pharyngitis and reduces risk of developing rheumatic fever. Clindamycin is effective if the patient is penicillin allergic. Oral corticosteroids, particularly single-dose dexamethasone, reduce severity and duration of symptoms.

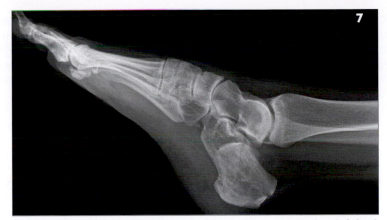

7 A 43-year-old female fell off a ladder and had severe pain in her left heel.
i. What does this radiograph demonstrate (7)?
ii. Is surgery necessary?

8 A 27-year-old male presented after being found unconscious outside someone's home. BP was 96/60 mmHg (12.8/8.0 kPa), P 128 bpm, RR 28/min, and T 35.6°C rectally. He had dilated pupils, conjunctival injection, and moved all extremities to sternal pressure stimulation. There was no external evidence of trauma. Laboratory studies included Na 132 mmol/l (132 mEq/l), Cl 102 mmol/l (102 mEq/l), K 3.1 mmol/l (3.1 mEq/l), CO_2 6 mmol/l (6 mEq/l), and glucose 7.0 mmol/l (126 mg/dl).

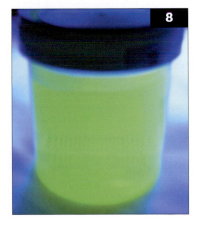

i. Your physician friend used an ultraviolet light to illuminate the patient's urine (8). What does this suggest?
ii. How should the patient be managed?

7 i. A calcaneus, or os calcis, fracture. The calcaneus is the most commonly fractured tarsal bone and plays a critical role in foot biomechanics and weight bearing. The mechanism of injury here is axial loading to the heel, which drives the talus down on the calcaneus. There are often associated fractures in the axial skeleton, including spine and other lower extremity fractures, which may need to be sought out. Pain, swelling, ecchymoses, and heel deformity are found on examination. Many classification systems exist for calcaneus fracture, describing an oblique, primary fracture line and multiple types of secondary fracture lines. Most calcaneus fractures are significantly displaced, and about 70% are intra-articular. Although plain radiographs may be adequate for evaluation, CT is often necessary.
ii. Operative versus nonoperative management for calcaneus fracture is controversial. Nondisplaced fractures may be managed conservatively with padding, ice, elevation, and no weight bearing until healed. Orthopedic consultation is important for all displaced os calcis fractures. Treatment goals of operative management are restoration of heel length, height, and hindfoot mechanical axis as well as realignment of the subtalar joint posterior facet. Multiple surgical techniques exist.

8 i. This unconscious young male has a large anion gap metabolic acidosis (anion gap = Na - (Cl + CO_2) = 132 - (102 + 6) = 24 [normal 8–12]). Remember causes using the mneumonic MUDPILES (Methanol or Metformin, Uremia, Diabetic ketoacidosis, Propylene glycol or Phenformin, Isoniazid or Iron, Lactic acidosis, Ethylene glycol or Ethanol, and Salicylates), which misses out cyanide and other rarities. Fluorescent urine is suggestive, as fluorescein is added to radiator antifreeze to help detect leaks, with ethylene glycol its main ingredient. It is ingested as a cheap alcohol substitute, accidentally or in suicide attempts. Ethylene glycol is metabolized by alcohol dehydrogenase to glycoaldehyde, then by aldehyde dehydrogenase to glycolic acid and other metabolites, producing profound acidosis. Early recognition of ingestion is difficult as initial metabolic disturbances may be minimal. An elevated osmolal gap (measured - calculated osmolality [2 times Na + BUN + glucose + EtOH] >10)* suggests unrecognized osmolar agents, including ethylene glycol. Urinalysis may show suggestive oxalate crystals.
ii. IV crystalloid resuscitation is necessary. Measure electrolytes, calcium, magnesium, and osmolality. Administer pyridoxine and thiamine, cofactors in ethylene glycol metabolism. Fomepizole is convenient, but expensive, therapy for both ethylene glycol and methanol poisoning. Oral or parenteral ethanol is effective and inexpensive, with weight-based titration to approximately 21.7 mmol/l (100 mg/dl) recommended. Hemodialysis is used in severe intoxication or renal insufficiency.
* [2 times Na + BUN/2.8 + glucose/18 + EtOH/4.6] in American units

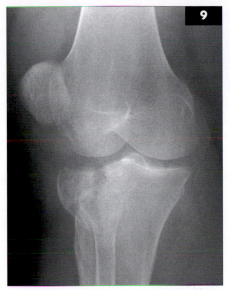

9 A 28-year-old male presented with a swollen, painful right knee after slipping on the ice 6 days ago. He cannot bear weight on his right lower extremity.
i. What does this radiograph show (9)?
ii. What is the treatment of choice?

10 A 25-year-old male presents with new-onset recurrent seizures. He is confused, diaphoretic, and incontinent of urine. BP is 244/140 mmHg (32.5/18.7 kPa), P 156 bpm, and T 39.2°C. A friend states that he abuses alcohol and may also use illicit drugs.
i. What do you think is going on?
ii. How should this patient be managed?

9 i. A lateral tibial plateau fracture. The tibial plateau is the most proximal part of the tibia, and fractures of this important load-bearing area affect range-of-motion, stability, and alignment. Careful evaluation is necessary for proper management. Tibial plateau fractures are usually due to valgus stress with axial load, often from falls or trauma from automobile bumpers. The lateral plateau is more commonly injured than the medial. The superficial nature of the knee means open fractures are common. Concomitant ligaments or meniscus injuries are frequent. Patients usually present with joint pain and effusion. Plain radiographs (multiple views) can usually recognize tibial plateau fractures. CT is often necessary to further characterize degree of tibial depression, displacement of fracture parts, and help plan orthopedic repair. MRI is excellent for recognition of meniscus or ligament injury. Arteriography may be indicated if popliteal artery injury is suspected.

ii. CT confirmed a surprising degree of tibial plateau depression and bony separation. Orthopedic consultation for surgical management is indicated. Immobilization is appropriate. Pain management and neurovascular monitoring, observing for popliteal artery occlusion due to unrecognized injury, is important.

10 i. This is a hyperadrenergic crisis, which has a short list of likely causes: cocaine or amphetamine toxicity, hyperthyroidism, pheochromocytoma, monamine-oxidase inhibitor interaction, as well as withdrawal from beta blockers, clonidine, or sedative-hypnotics (e.g. alcohol). In this case excessive cocaine use was suspected and felt to be the likely etiology.

ii. Benzodiazepines (e.g. lorazepam) in high doses are the drugs of choice in this situation. They directly enhance GABA-mediated neuronal inhibition and terminate seizures in most cocaine intoxications. (Also the right choice for sedative-hypnotic withdrawal.) External cooling of fever is important. Refrain from beta blockers in acute cocaine intoxication to avoid unopposed alpha adrenergic receptor stimulation. Neuroimaging to exclude intracranial hemorrhage may be important, as well as ECG and biomarker studies to evaluate for cardiac injury.

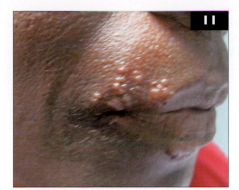

11 This 34-year-old female presented with a painful rash on her right upper lip (**11**) that she associated with use of a new lip balm.
i. What is the rash, and did the lip balm cause it?
ii. How should it be treated?

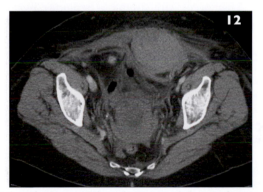

12 A 54-year-old female presented with severe abdominal pain, which had been progressive over several hours. She had nausea with vomiting twice in the day prior and a normal bowel movement last night. She had recently started a new heart medication, but did not know its name. BP was 136/84 mmHg (18.1/11.2 kPa), P 96 bpm and irregular, RR 18/min, and T 37.8°C. Her left mid-abdomen was very tender with a palpable firm mass just left of the midline. An abdominal CT scan was done (**12**).
i. What do you think is the culprit medication?
ii. How should the patient be managed?

11 i. Herpes labialis, or cold sores, an infection of the lips, mouth, or gums with herpes simplex virus (HSV). Primary infections are frequently asymptomatic and may be caused by HSV-1 or HSV-2. Prodromal symptoms include local itching, burning, tingling, or skin hypersensitivity. A local, painful vesicular rash on an erythematous base occurs, with blister rupture and crusting occurring over time. Diagnosis is made by appearance or by cultures from the lesion. There may be local lymphadenopathy. Recurrent cold sores are common and may be triggered by sun exposure, fever, stress, or menstruation, among other causes. The first episode may last up to 2–3 weeks. The lip balm likely did not cause this problem.
ii. Treatment should begin at symptom onset for best results. Several topical antiviral agents (e.g. acyclovir cream) reduce symptoms and duration of outbreak. New, high-dose, 1-day oral regimens using famciclovir or valacyclovir are also effective, and these medications in lower doses can be taken daily to reduce the reactivation rate. Other topical and oral therapies exist.

12 i. Coumadin, an anticoagulant, was recently added to the patient's medications (she was in atrial fibrillation). Her prothrombin time was 44.9 seconds (normal 10.0–12.6 seconds) with an INR of 4.5. The patient has a rectus sheath hematoma, which is uncommon and frequently misdiagnosed. They are usually traumatic, a result of bleeding from damage to superior or inferior epigastric arteries or from rectus muscle tears. They occur with strenuous activities, but occasionally simply with coughing or vomiting, the likely trigger in this overly anticoagulated patient. Diagnosis is often clinical, with a palpable, tender, nonpulsatile, firm mass in the rectus sheath area. Obesity may complicate examination. Increased pain with tensing abdominal muscles by raising the head or shoulders while lying down (Carnett's sign) is very suggestive of abdominal musculature problems. Periumbilical ecchymoses (Cullen's sign) and flank bruising (Grey Turner sign) are associated with abdominal wall hemorrhage. Ultrasound is usually diagnostic and can characterize the mass.
ii. Conservative measures, including rest, analgesics, local ice, abdominal wall compression, and management of predisposing conditions, are usually sufficient. Rapid reversal of anticoagulation should be considered, particularly with expansion, associated significant anemia, or hemodynamic instability. Fluid resuscitation and transfusion may occasionally be necessary.

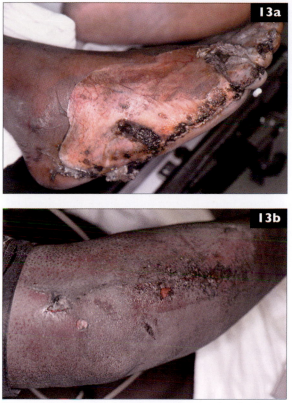

13 A 47-year-old electrical worker was burned when his basket crane accidently engaged with high-voltage electrical wires.
i. What do these burns represent in terms of amount of injury (**13a, b**)?
ii. How should he be managed?

14 A 29-year-old male was found unconscious outside. He had a BP of 86/52 mmHg (11.5/6.9 kPa), P 52 bpm, RR 8/min, T 36.8°C, and pinpoint pupils.
i. What is the likely diagnosis?
ii. What tests and therapies are necessary here?

13 i. Severe electrical burns from a high-voltage, alternating-current industrial line (can carry >100,000 volts). Electrical damage to tissue is related to voltage, current strength, tissue resistance, and duration of source contact. Blood vessels, nerves, and muscles have low resistance, much less than fat, bone, or skin (unless wet skin!). Direct contact electrical burns cause thermoelectric injury at the entrance and exit of the electron flow, but also along its path in proportion to electrical resistance. Alteration of muscle function is more related to current, with skeletal muscle tetany (including respiratory muscles) at as little as 20 milliamps and ventricular fibrillation at >50 milliamps.

ii. The first priority is safe removal from the source, being careful not to create other victims. Ensuring ventilation and addressing arrhythmias (e.g. ventricular fibrillation) comes next. Provide adequate pain management. Finally, evaluate contact and ground sites injury, along with the electrical path traversed between sites. Underlying tissue injury is often more severe than apparent. CBC, creatine kinase, serum myoglobin, electrolytes, urinalysis, and renal function studies are important. An ECG is appropriate. Utilize other imaging modalities as needed. Volume resuscitate with appropriate hemodynamic monitoring. Fasciotomy may be necessary if clinical evidence or measurements suggest compartment syndrome.

14 i. The hypotension, bradycardia, hypoventilation, and pinpoint pupils are most suggestive of opiate overdose.

ii. A search for needle tracks or recent injection sites, as well as a clothing inventory for evidence of narcotics or paraphernalia, may help confirm the diagnosis. Prescription oral narcotic abuse is increasing worldwide. The only diagnostic test appropriate at this time is therapeutic challenge with naloxone, starting with 1–2 mg parenterally. Improvement in vital signs and level of consciousness is diagnostic. Response may be suboptimal in polysubstance overdose. Urine toxicology screening may help, but many synthetic opiates are not recognized with standard urine drug panels.

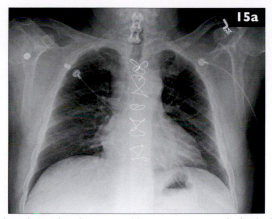

15 A 61-year-old male with a history of hypertension and alcohol abuse allegedly fell about 4 hours ago. He was light-headed and weak, with pleuritic left chest pain. BP was 96/60 mmHg (12.8/8.0 kPa) and P 136 bpm. He seemed tender in his left lateral lower chest wall and upper abdomen.
i. What does his chest radiograph show (**15a**)?
ii. What other imaging is indicated?
iii. How should the patient be managed?

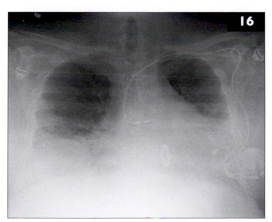

16 A 64-year-old female presented after a short syncopal episode and her ECG showed a slow bradycardia with atrial fibrillation.
i. What important diagnosis is suggested by the chest radiograph (**16**)?
ii. What is the appropriate therapy?

15 i. Minimal evidence of injury, but suggests previous sternotomy and cervical spine surgery, which the patient did not initially mention. There are no visible rib fractures, but chest radiography will frequently miss these as well as other significant underlying injuries. On a subtle note, his gastric bubble may be slightly displaced medially.

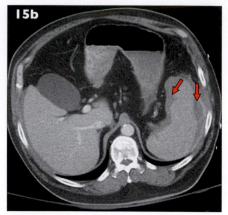

ii. Immediate ultrasound FAST examination, or contrasted abdominal CT imaging if hemodynamics improve. CT revealed a significant splenic injury with a large amount of surrounding blood (**15b**, arrows).

iii. Aggressive crystalloid volume resuscitation along with CBC, coagulation studies, electrolytes, and type and crossmatch for several units of blood. The patient remained hemodynamically unstable despite large volumes of crystalloid and blood, and he required emergency splenectomy.

16 i. This is a fine example of Twiddler's syndrome, a rare cause of permanent pacemaker malfunction. In this disorder the pacemaker generator is accidentally or deliberately spun in a roomy, subcutaneous pocket. Pacemaker leads are dislodged and loop near or around the pulse generator. Failure of electrical capture and sensing ensues, with frequent symptomatic bradyarrhythmias. With continued manipulation, pacemaker leads are further extracted from the heart, sometimes stimulating the phrenic nerve with rhythmic diaphragmatic contractions or pectoral muscles with chest and arm twitching. The chest radiograph demonstrates looping of electrode leads around or near the pulse generator, occasionally with lead fracture. Electrodes may also be malpositioned in relation to appropriate cardiac implantation. ECG may show an intrinsic underlying rhythm with pacemaker spikes indicating failure to sense and/or capture. Twiddler's syndrome may be fatal if the underlying cardiac rhythm is nonperfusing.

ii. Emergency transcutaneous pacing may be necessary to provide a perfusing rhythm, with transvenous pacing only if this fails. Immediate cardiology consultation is necessary for removal and replacement of the permanent pacemaker, hopefully in a tighter tissue pocket. Psychiatric evaluation may be necessary in selected patients.

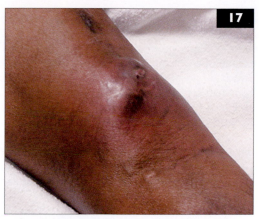

17 A 53-year-old male presented with pain and swelling at his hemodialysis fistula site (**17**). He denied any trauma other than due to normal needle access for dialysis and he had no fever or other systemic complaints.
i. What is this common complication of hemodialysis access?
ii. Can this vascular access be saved?

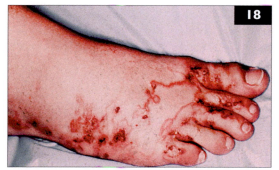

18 A 27-year-old male presented after an extended vacation to the Dominican Republic. He had this very itchy, red rash on his foot (**18**).
i. What is your diagnosis?
ii. How do you treat it?

17 i. Infectious complications of vascular access remain a major cause of morbidity and mortality in hemodialysis patients. This patient has alarming evidence of infection. The immune system is quite suppressed in renal insufficiency, with occult infection common. Lack of erythema, purulent discharge, or significant tenderness is common early in vascular access infection, making delayed recognition common. Primary arteriovenous fistulas have the lowest rates of infection, while indwelling catheters have the highest. Infection accounts for about 15% of all deaths in this patient population, with about 25% of these due to vascular access infectious complications.

ii. IV broad-spectrum antibiotics are required to cover *Staphylococcus aureus* as well as a large number of other potential culprit organisms. Surgical drainage and access removal was required in this case, as is usually necessary with extensive infection.

18 i. Cutaneous larva migrans, a common tropically acquired dermatitis, which might present anywhere in the world due to widespread travel. It is an erythematous, serpiginous, pruritic eruption caused by skin penetration of various nematode parasites. The parasites pass from animal feces to moist, sandy soil where larvae develop and penetrate the stratum corneum. These larvae lack the enzymes needed to invade the dermis in the accidental human host and are condemned to migrate in the epidermis. Local inflammatory changes cause the dermatitis. The typical patient has tropical or subtropical exposure to warm sandy soil, particularly barefoot beachgoers. Erythematous, slightly elevated, meandering, 2–3 mm wide tunnels track up to several cm from the penetration sites. Systemic signs are rare. The rash is usually on distal lower extremities, but may appear on any exposed skin. The most common etiology is *Ancylostoma braziliense* (dog and cat hookworm), but other hookworms and, rarely, other parasites may cause cutaneous larva migrans. Skin biopsy of the leading edge of a tract may show a larva in a burrow.

ii. The condition is self-limiting, but most patients want rapid, effective therapy. A topical 10–15% suspension of thiabendazole will decrease pruritis within 1–2 days and resolve dermatitis in a week or so. For widespread cutaneous larva migrans or failure of topical therapy, oral albendazole, mebendazole, ivermectin, or thiabendazole will be effective. Liquid nitrogen cryotherapy to the proximal end of the larval burrow has been used. Oral antibiotics are indicated in secondary bacterial infections.

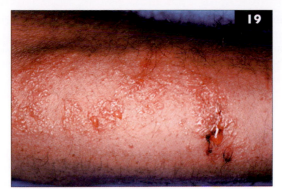

19 A 27-year-old male presented with an itchy rash (**19**). He was an avid outdoorsman.
i. What is this rash?
ii. How should it be treated?

20 A 34-year-old male was involved in a fist fight while intoxicated last night and presented with pain and swelling on the dorsal and radial side of his left hand.
i. What problem is shown on the radiograph (**20**)?
ii. How should it be managed?

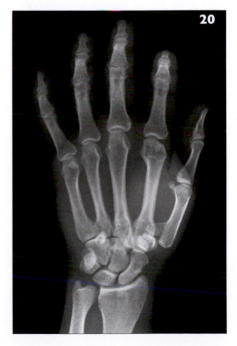

19 i. This is a fine example of an allergic contact dermatitis, occurring here due to exposure to members of the plant genus *Toxicodendron* such as poison ivy, poison oak, and, less commonly, poison sumac. These plants produce the skin-irritating oil urushiol, which can cause a severe type IV delayed hypersensitivity reaction. Exposure is typically topical, although severe allergic reactions can occur with inhalation of burning plant material. The rash typically begins 12–24 hours after exposure and lasts 2–3 weeks. The characteristic rash is a linear, erythematous, edematous, pruritic, weeping dermatitis with vesicles.

ii. Classic preventive strategies include wearing long sleeves, pants, and vinyl gloves. Treatment of any contact dermatitis begins with attempts to remove the offending sensitizing agents, usually with soap and water. Several commercially available creams are marketed to remove or prevent penetration of urushiol into the skin. Published data on these remedies are limited and conflicting. Topical corticosteroids may be adequate for very small areas of rash, but systemic corticosteroids (e.g. prednisone 1–2 mg/kg/day) are usually necessary, sometimes for as long as 10–14 days. Antihistamines are helpful for pruritis.

20 i. There is an intra-articular fracture at the ulnar base of the first carpo-metacarpal joint, termed a Bennett's fracture. Early diagnosis and proper management is necessary to avoid loss of thumb function, as this joint is important for pinch and opposition. Inappropriate management may lead to an unstable arthritic joint with loss of motion and chronic pain. The injury generally occurs when an axial load is applied to a partially flexed thumb. The critical volar oblique ligament avulses a piece of bone and pull from the abductor pollicis muscles frequently leads to progressive displacement. Pain and swelling occur at the thumb base and gentle valgus stress usually confirms instability.

ii. Closed reduction and thumb spica cast immobilization is effective in the management of some Bennett's fractures, but more than 1 mm of articular incongruity is an indication for operative intervention. Even with successful reduction and thumb casting, serial radiographs are necessary, as strong pull from the abductor pollicis muscles often leads to delayed displacement. Reduction with internal fixation is usually required for displaced Bennett's fractures, which may be done open or closed. Open reduction was necessary in this case.

21 A 43-year-old male had AIDS and presented with this facial swelling (**21**), which had developed over the past week. This was not his first time with this swelling. He was off all of his medications.

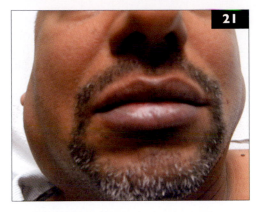

i. What is the problem here?
ii. What treatment does he require?

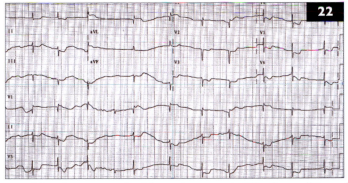

22 A 79-year-old male presented with weakness and difficulty walking, along with multiple episodes of nausea and vomiting. He denied chest pain or shortness of breath. He had a history of COPD and atrial fibrillation, for which he took prednisone, nebulized albuterol treatments, and digoxin. BP was 104/50 mmHg (13.9/6.7 kPa), with an irregular P of 60 bpm, RR 18/min, T 37.8°C, and P_{ox} 95%. On examination, he had clear lungs, an irregular S_1 and S_2, jugular venous distension, and bipedal edema.

i. What does this ECG suggest (**22**)?
ii. How should the patient be managed?

21 i. This is impressive bilateral parotid swelling. The parotid glands are small exocrine glands that produce saliva. Infectious and autoimmune causes are the most common precipitants of acute parotitis. If unilateral, salivary duct stones must be considered. Acute bacterial parotitis is commonly caused by *Staphylococcus aureus*, but studies show mixed infections are frequent. Viral etiologies include mumps most commonly, but here HIV is the precipitant.
ii. HIV therapy is the treatment of choice in this case and may lead to rapid improvement.

22 i. Digoxin toxicity. The ECG shows atrial fibrillation, bradycardia, and downsloping ST segment depressions in leads V_2–V_6. Digoxin, a cardiac glycoside, inhibits membrane-bound Na/K ATPase, secondarily elevating sarcoplasmic membrane calcium and increasing cardiac contractility. The most common cause of digoxin toxicity is associated hypokalemia; it also occurs more frequently with advanced age and renal insufficiency. Multiple medications reduce digoxin clearance, particularly macrolide antibiotics, calcium channel blockers, and quinidine. Symptoms of digoxin toxicity are mainly gastrointestinal (e.g. vomiting, diarrhea), cardiac (e.g. palpitations, heart failure exacerbation) and CNS (e.g. weakness, confusion). ECG changes include bradycardia, PR prolongation, QT shortening, downsloping ST segment depression in precordial leads, premature ventricular contractions, and rare rhythms (e.g. reciprocating ventricular tachycardia or paroxysmal atrial tachycardia with atrioventricular block).
ii. Digoxin levels correlate poorly with toxicity, particularly with chronic poisoning. (Steady-state levels are delayed several hours after oral dosing.) For acute digoxin overdose, activated charcoal will reduce absorption. Treat hypokalemia and hypomagnesemia (which exacerbate digoxin toxicity). Manage hyperkalemia (due to Na/K ATPase dysfunction) in the usual manner, except avoid calcium (possibly proarrhythmic in digoxin toxicity). An effective digoxin-specific antibody is available. Indications include postdistribution serum digoxin levels >6.4 nmol/l (5 ng/ml), as well as suspected toxicity with hyperkalemia, ventricular arrhythmias, high-degree atrioventricular block, rapidly progressive signs or symptoms of toxicity, cardiac arrest, cardiogenic shock, or acute ingestion of massive quantities of digoxin. This patient's level was 7.2 nmol/l (5.6 ng/ml) and he responded rapidly to digoxin immunotherapy.

23 A 48-year-old male presented after a sudden, severe headache that caused a brief episode of syncope. A few hours later he was neurologically perfect, but with diffuse headache and mild neck stiffness.

i. What does this head CT image suggest (**23a**)?

ii. What treatment is indicated?

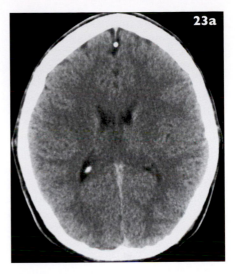

24 A 53-year-old Vietnamese male presented with a mild fever and these skin changes (**24**). What is going on here?

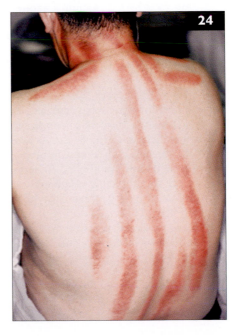

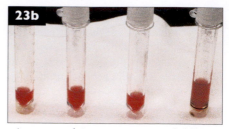

23 i. The history suggests SAH (bleeding between brain pial and arachnoid membranes), but here CT imaging is non-diagnostic. Trauma is the most common SAH etiology, so ascertain if significant head injury occurred with the syncopal event. Cerebral aneurysm is the most common etiology in nontraumatic SAH (two-thirds), with arteriovenous malformation second (most common childhood etiology). Nontraumatic SAH typically presents as a sudden, severe, diffuse headache reaching peak intensity within seconds to minutes, often with syncope, vomiting, meningeal signs, various neurologic deficits, and seizures. Sentinel or warning leak headache occurs in 30–50% of nontraumatic SAH, usually within the 2 weeks preceding rupture. Embolic events and mass effect from compression of adjacent structures are other SAH presentations. Complications include stroke, rebleeding, cerebral artery vasospasm, hydrocephalus, and seizures. CT is usually diagnostic for SAH early after presentation, although a few have normal CT, requiring lumbar puncture for confirmation (**23b**). CT or MRA helps define the bleeding site and presence of aneurysms.

ii. Attention to ABC is important. Major bleeds with altered mental status may require endotracheal intubation for airway protection and support. Head of bed elevation to 30–45°, calcium channel blocker (nicardipine) to reduce cerebral vasospasm, judicious saline infusions, and antiepileptic medications are standard therapies. Prompt neurosurgical consultation is important. Mortality is high in SAH, with a third or more dying within 30 days. Many survivors have significant neurologic deficits.

24 This is an example of skin changes due to coining, or cao gio (pronounced gow yaw), a form of alternative medicine most commonly practiced in Southeast Asia. In this culture it is thought to create a path for release of 'bad wind', believed to be the cause of illness. Coining is advocated for treatment of various illnesses including colds, headaches, and fever. Cupping is a similar practice in the Chinese culture, where heated cups are applied to acupuncture sites or areas of pain. As the cups cool, skin suction with resultant bruising occurs. Moxibustion involves the application of heat generated by burning small bundles of herbs, or moxa, to targeted areas, thus promoting flow of blood and vital energy. Many Eastern cultures have similar practices with various techniques and names. Complications of these treatments are rare and mostly involve thermal burns and ecchymoses. The skin changes are occasionally reported as child or elder abuse.

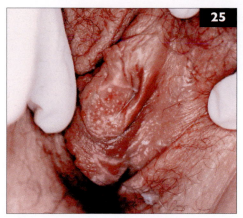

25 A 24-year-old female presented with these painless sores in her vaginal area (25). She denied trauma, but did admit to recent unprotected sex with a new partner.
i. What are these sores?
ii. How is the condition confirmed and treated?

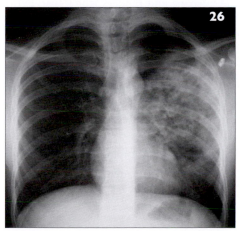

26 A 34-year-old male patient presented with new onset, generalized, tonic–clonic seizures. He was on multiple unknown medications to treat pneumonia. Repeated doses of lorazepam as well as loading doses of phenytoin and phenobarbital failed to control the seizures.
i. Does this chest radiograph suggest the likely problem in this patient (26)?
ii. What treatment is likely to resolve this seizure activity?

25 i. Chancres, painless local erosions due to primary syphilis. This infectious lesion appears about 3 weeks after direct exposure to *Treponema pallidum*, a gram-negative spirochete. Firm, painless, ulcerative lesions occur in areas of local sexual contact, primarily the penis, vagina, mouth, and anus. Chancres can heal spontaneously without treatment in 1–6 weeks.

ii. Dark field microscopy of fluid from primary or secondary syphilis will reveal spirochetes. Rapid plasma reagin (RPR) and Venereal Disease Research Laboratory (VDRL) blood tests are useful to diagnose syphilis, but both suffer from frequent false-positive results. Confirmatory testing with *T. pallidum* hemagglutination assay and fluorescent treponemal antibody absorption tests are recommended, although these may be falsely positive in other treponemal diseases (e.g. yaws). An ELISA for *T. pallidum* also exists. Penicillin remains the therapy of first choice for all manifestations of syphilis. Chancre may be treated with a single dose of benzathine penicillin, with doxycycline or tetracycline used if severe penicillin allergy. Azithromycin is no longer recommended, as resistance has developed for *T. pallidum*.

26 i. The radiograph shows a diffuse left upper lobe infiltrate suggesting, among other things, pulmonary tuberculosis. In the clinical setting of uncontrolled seizure activity despite multiple antiepileptic agents, isoniazid toxicity must be strongly considered. Ingestion of >30 mg/kg of isoniazid may cause seizures refractory to aggressive conventional therapy. Isoniazid is a common antituberculosis medication that combines with pyridoxine and renders it inactive. Pyridoxine is required to produce GABA in the brain, and GABA depletion greatly increases susceptibility to seizures. High anion gap metabolic acidosis and coma are other presentations of isoniazid toxicity.

ii. In suspected isoniazid-related seizures, pyridoxine should be administered in a dose equivalent to the suspected amount of isoniazid ingested. When the quantity is unknown, give 5 g of pyridoxine IV over 5–10 minutes. There should be a low threshold for giving pyridoxine in suspected isoniazid toxicity with seizures. It should also be considered in any refractory seizure activity. This patient was given pyridoxine (5 g IV), with prompt resolution. On awakening, he admitted to overdosing on his tuberculosis medications as a suicide attempt.

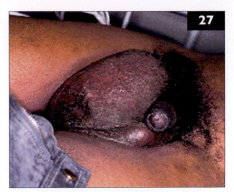

27 A 32-year-old male presented with recurrent scrotal swelling (27), which was suddenly much more painful than usual. He could get the intermittent scrotal swelling to go away completely in the past, but not today.
i. What is the main differential diagnosis in this patient?
ii. What evaluation and treatment strategy is indicated?

28 A 23-year-old athlete injured his knee during a basketball game. It was very swollen, painful, and difficult to examine.
i. What does this knee radiograph show, and what does it suggest (28)?
ii. What should be done?

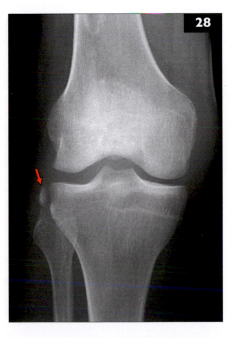

27 i. Unilateral scrotal swelling can be due to testicular disorders including orchitis, malignancy, injury, and torsion. Surrounding structures may be involved with such problems as varicocele, hydrocele, and epididymitis. Here, indirect inguinal hernia is likely. Although often uncomfortable, severe pain unlike previous episodes may suggest intestinal ischemia due to strangulation. Symptoms of bowel obstruction are also common.

ii. Treatment depends on the suspected etiology. If testicular or related to surrounding structures, ultrasound evaluation will dictate treatment. Here, the recurrent nature, massive swelling, and asymptomatic intervals make indirect inguinal hernia likely. Bowel sounds may be appreciated on direct auscultation. Plain radiographs may reveal bowel loops in the scrotal sac. CT can confirm, but is usually unnecessary. A surgeon should be consulted if there is suspicion of strangulation or evidence of peritonitis. If unavailable, consider manual hernia reduction. Procedural sedation, supine Trendelenburg position, and constant encompassing pressure to slowly reduce intestinal loops back into the abdomen may be effective. Skilled operators may find ultrasound assists in reduction. A theoretical concern is return of necrotic bowel to the abdominal cavity, which rarely occurs because resultant swelling of dead tissue makes reduction difficult. Successful reduction is marked by loss of scrotal swelling, along with pain resolution. Evidence of peritonitis, ongoing pain after hernia manipulation, failure of reduction, or suspected ischemic bowel dictates prompt surgical involvement (also eventually necessary for definitive surgical repair).

28 i. Segond fracture, a type of vertical avulsion injury of the lateral tibeal plateau (**28**, arrow). Segond fracture occurs in association with tears of the anterior cruciate ligament (75–100%), with concomitant injury of the medial meniscus (66–75%), along with soft tissue injuries to the posterior knee. This injury is usually the result of varus stress combined with internal rotation to the knee. A more rare reverse Segond fracture has also been described. Here, a medial tibial avulsion is pulled off by the medial collateral ligament and is associated with posterior cruciate ligament injury, medial meniscus tears, and soft tissue damage. Both of these fractures are typically quite small and best seen on anterior/posterior radiographs, but may require CT or MRI for visualization.

ii. This fracture implies severe ligamentous and internal injury to the knee. A careful neurovascular examination with ongoing monitoring is indicated. Prompt orthopedic consultation is appropriate for further evaluation and surgical repair.

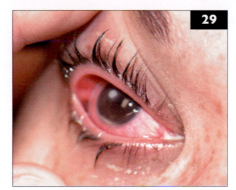

29 This 26-year-old had been using extended-wear contacts and developed eye redness with mild pain over the last few days (29).
i. What is this clinical finding?
ii. What management is indicated?

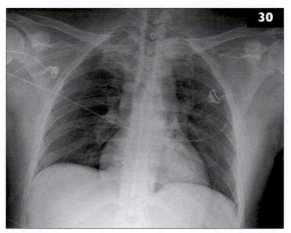

30 A 32-year-old male presented after a short episode of syncope and felt quite short of breath. He had knee surgery 3 weeks ago and was still in a cast. He had no other previous medical problems. BP was 96/60 mmHg (12.8/8.0 kPa) with P 128 bpm, RR 26/min, temperature 38°C, and P_{ox} 94%.
i. What is the likely diagnosis, based on this chest radiograph (30)?
ii. How should the diagnosis be confirmed?
iii. What is appropriate treatment?

29 i. Hypopyon, an accumulation of WBCs in the eye's anterior chamber. Hypopyon is actually sterile pus, occurring secondary to toxin release rather than due directly to infectious agents. In this patient, a small corneal ulcer secondary to prolonged contact use caused the hypopyon. It may also be secondary to penetrating eye trauma and infection, as well as neoplastic (e.g. leukemia) and inflammatory (e.g. Behcet's disease) causes. Hypopyon is a sign of anterior uveitis and is usually accompanied by conjunctival injection. A careful work-up is important if the cause is not obvious. Uveitis is a significant cause of blindness if not managed properly.

ii. Treatment is etiology specific. An associated keratitis requires aggressive anti-biotic (e.g. moxifloxacin) or antiviral drops, as indicated. Other etiologies are treated after ophthalmology consultation, often with corticosteroids and, occasionally, other immunosuppressive therapy.

30 i. This essentially normal radiograph raises suspicion for hemodynamically significant pulmonary emboli. Most are complications of lower extremity deep venous thrombophlebitis. Increased age, trauma, immobilization, pregnancy, recent surgery, multiple medical diseases (e.g. malignancy, heart failure), vasculitis, disorders of coagulation and fibrinolysis, and certain medications (e.g. estrogen) are the main risk factors. Over 20% have no risk factor identified. Main symptoms of pulmonary emboli are chest pain, dyspnea, hemoptysis, and syncope. Physical examination shows nonspecific findings, but tachycardia, rales, and clinical evidence of deep venous thrombophlebitis are important hints.

ii. Diagnosis of pulmonary embolism is frequently difficult and requires inclusion in the differential diagnosis of chest pain or shortness of breath. Hypoxia is variable and does not correlate with severity. Chest radiographs and ECG are rarely diagnostic. D-dimer is usually elevated in intravascular clotting. In low clinical risk cases, normal D-dimer makes pulmonary emboli unlikely. Cardiac ultrasound findings include dilated right ventricle (RV normally two-thirds diameter of LV) and septal shift to the left. High-resolution CT angiography has excellent sensitivity and specificity for clinically significant pulmonary emboli and is the definitive imaging modality of choice. A ventilation–perfusion lung scan is less sensitive and specific.

iii. Hypoxia contributes greatly to mortality, so supplemental oxygen, and even mechanical ventilation, may be necessary. Anticoagulation with unfractionated or low molecular weight heparin should be initiated immediately if not contra-indicated. Thrombolytic therapy is used in hemodynamic compromise or un-resolved hypoxia, but lacks research evidence of mortality reduction. Surgical clot removal, as well as mechanical transvenous clot fragmentation and extraction, may be life saving in extreme cases.

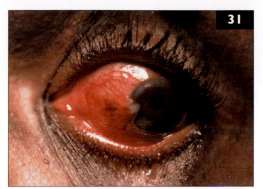

31 A 44-year-old male presented with a few hours of left eye itching and redness (**31**), without history of trauma.
i. What is the problem?
ii. Does the patient need treatment?

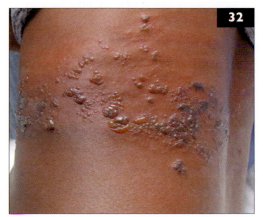

32 A 46-year-old female presented after 4 days of severe, left lower back pain and 1 day of a red, blistered rash in that area (**32**). She used a heating pad on it last night without relief.
i. What is the rash?
ii. How should it be managed?

31 i. Pterygium, a very common degenerative condition of the conjunctiva presenting as an elevated fibrovascular proliferation. It usually originates from the medial canthal area and over several years extends onto the corneal surface. Risk factors for pterygium are related to prolonged ultraviolet light exposure, with some genetic predisposition. Most cases are asymptomatic, but redness, swelling, itching, or blurred vision may occur. A pinguecula is similar to a pterygium, but does not extend onto the cornea. Rarely, malignancy or trauma may cause a similar appearance.

ii. Treatment of symptomatic pterygium includes over-the-counter artificial tears or lubricating ointments, with topical corticosteroids occasionally used short term for inflammatory exacerbations. Surgical excision may be needed for cosmetic reasons, functional discomfort, or vision issues. Radiation therapy and topical antineoplastic agents (e.g. mitomycin C) are used in rare circumstances.

32 i. Shingles (herpes zoster), complicated by slight thermal burn (heating pad). Herpes zoster results from varicella virus reactivation from any dorsal nerve root. It occurs at any age, but more commonly if elderly or immunosuppressed. Shingles may present as burning, hyperesthetic, dermatomal pain for several days before rash eruption. Fever and headache are sometimes associated. Erythematous rash appears with multiple grouped vesicles spread irregularly through a dermatomal distribution. Most common on the trunk, it may involve the eye (sometimes permanent damage) or ear (vertigo and hearing loss). Herpes simplex virus occasionally produces similar dermatomal rash. Tzanck smear, varicella specific IgM antibody titer, PCR, or viral culture may help in difficult cases.

ii. Aggressive pain management is appropriate, often requiring narcotics. Topical calamine lotions can soothe. Antiviral drugs (e.g. acyclovir) are most effective if started within 72 hours of rash appearance. They shorten primary infection duration, but probably not the incidence of postherpetic neuralgia, a chronic residual dermatomal pain syndrome. Immunocompromised hosts with shingles should receive IV acyclovir to reduce complications. Corticosteroid use is controversial, but may improve lesion healing time and early pain, while not reducing incidence of postherpetic neuralgia. Capsaicin cream is useful to relieve pain after lesions have crusted. Gabapentin may reduce pain in postherpetic neuralgia. A recent live-attenuated vaccine (Zostavax) reduces herpes zoster incidence by half as well as the rate of postherpetic neuralgia.

33 An 18-year-old female presented from the dentist's office with acute confusion. She had no known medical problems and was simply getting a couple of dental extractions. She had blue lips and fingertips.
i. What does this presentation suggest?
ii. How should the patient be treated?

34 A 26-year-old male hurt his right middle finger when he jammed it playing baseball. He presented with a swollen, tender middle finger at the distal interphalangeal joint, which was slightly flexed and with pain on any range of motion.
i. What does this radiograph suggest (34)?
ii. How should he be managed?

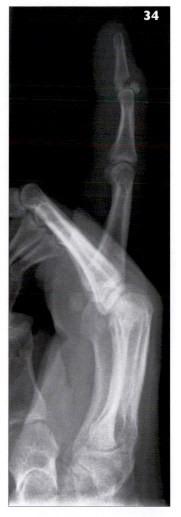

33 i. Cyanosis and confusion suggests methemoglobinemia, probably caused by local anesthetic. Each hemoglobin molecule contains four polypeptide chains associated with four heme groups, each having an iron molecule normally in the ferrous (Fe^{2+}) state. Oxidative stressors convert iron from ferrous to ferric (Fe^{3+}) state, creating methemoglobin, which is incapable of oxygen transport. Agents inflicting oxidative stress include many local anesthetics (e.g. lidocaine), various nitrites and nitrates, some antimalarials (e.g. chloroquine), some antibiotics (e.g. sulfonamides), along with several other medications and environmental agents. Significant methemoglobinemia (25–50%) presents with dyspnea, palpitations, chest pain, and various neurologic symptoms (headache, weakness, confusion, and seizures). Cyanosis occurs with levels >15–20%, but may be relatively asymptomatic. Pulse oximetry is inaccurate with methemoglobin, which absorbs light wavelengths also absorbed by deoxyhemoglobin and oxyhemoglobin. Measuring methemoglobin levels requires a multiple wavelength co-oximeter.

ii. Recognition of methemoglobinemia should trigger therapy. Dermal and gastrointestinal decontamination may be appropriate. Supplemental oxygen does not increase transported oxygen significantly. Low levels (e.g. 10%) may need only observation. Methylene blue is the main antidote for symptomatic methemoglobinemia, with initial dose 1–2 g IV. Response should occur within 20 minutes. Avoid methylene blue in glucose-6-phosphate dehydrogenase deficiency (hemolysis). It may be ineffective with ongoing oxidative stress or in patients lacking certain methemoglobin reductase enzymes. Hyperbaric oxygen and/or RBC exchange transfusion are rarely necessary.

34 i. This patient has a proximal dorsal distal phalanx fracture with intra-articular involvement, often termed a mallet finger fracture. The fingertip rests in an abnormally flexed position due to loss of extension at the distal interphalangeal joint. Frequently, the extensor tendon is pulled off, with minimal or no fracture. The typical mechanism of mallet finger injury is forced flexion of a finger held in extension, a common sports injury.

ii. Surprisingly, whether bony or tendinous, almost all mallet finger injuries can be treated with dorsal splinting in full extension for 6–8 weeks with excellent results. The associated fracture does not change the prognosis or, usually, require surgical repair. Patient adherence to continuous splint wearing for the entire period is important. Orthopedic reduction with Krischner wire fixation is rarely necessary.

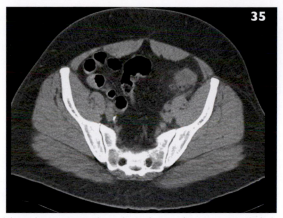

35 A 44-year-old male presented with 2 days of increasing left lower abdominal pain along with nausea and some watery diarrhea. There was no travel history, recent fever, or other complaints. On physical examination he had normal vital signs, but moderate tenderness in the left lower quadrant of his abdomen.
i. What does this CT image suggest (35)?
ii. How should the patient be managed?

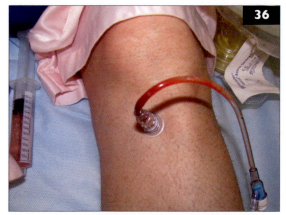

36 A 53-year-old female presented with this finding (36).
i. What is this?
ii. What can be infused through it?

35 i. Inflammation around sigmoid diverticuli, suggesting acute diverticulitis. Diverticula are small mucosal herniations protruding through intestinal layers along natural openings created by nutrient vessels. Most are colonic, mainly sigmoid. Diverticulitis is inflammation of one or more diverticula. Pathogenesis is unclear, but probably due to obstruction by fecal material or undigested food. Diverticular distension with bacterial overgrowth and microperforations ensue. Frank perforation, abscess, and fistula formation are the main complications. Presentations include pain, mostly in the left lower abdomen, along with constipation or diarrhea, nausea, vomiting, flatulence, and bloating. Local abdominal tenderness and fever are common. With abscess formation, a mass may be palpated. Free perforation may lead to diffuse peritonitis. Simple diverticulitis is a clinical diagnosis with laboratory tests and radiographic imaging most useful in unclear cases.

ii. Uncomplicated diverticulitis can have outpatient treatment, with light diet and oral broad-spectrum antimicrobial therapy covering typical bowel flora. Metronidazole combined with a fluoroquinolone (e.g. ciprofloxacin) or trimethoprim–sulfamethoxazole, as well as monotherapy with amoxicillin/ clavulanate, is commonly used, with treatment for 7–10 days. Hospitalization and IV antibiotics are necessary for complicated cases, including patients with immunocompromise, systemic signs of infection, peritonitis, severe pain, substantial abscess, suspected perforation, and those who cannot obtain or keep down medications. Surgical consultation is frequently important in these patients. Percutaneous abscess drainage is often effective. Recurrent diverticulitis may require elective partial colectomy.

36 i. An intraosseous needle, a commercial vascular access often inserted using a drill device. Intraosseous access is a life-saving technique for patients with cardiovascular instability when conventional intravenous lines are not rapidly successful. This is a popular emergency technique in pediatric patients, but recent military experience and device improvement has increased its use in all unstable patients. Common insertion sites include proximal tibia, distal femoral condyle, and proximal humeral head at the greater tuberosity. Novice device users with various battery-operated needle drivers have high success rates, usually completing access in <20 seconds. Main complications in adults are infusion device dislodgement and extravasation.

ii. Infusion of fluids by this route (essentially all medications and blood products) compares favorably with IV access in terms of infusion rates and delivery to the central circulation. Intraosseous access is probably underutilized or inserted late in clinical situations where it may be life saving.

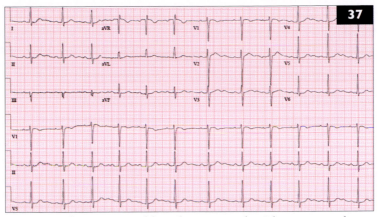

37 A very muscular 26-year-old male presented with acute weakness in his extremities, lower more than upper, to the point that he could not stand. He stated that he had intermittent similar weakness, although never this bad, after heavy exercise since adolescence. He seemed very nonchalant, and you became concerned about malingering.
i. Does his ECG make you change your mind (37)?
ii. How should the patient be managed?

38 A 42-year-old male presented with these hand findings (38), which became worse over several days. He had experienced this problem before, and some cream took care of it last time.
i. What is this problem, and what has caused it?
ii. How should it be treated?

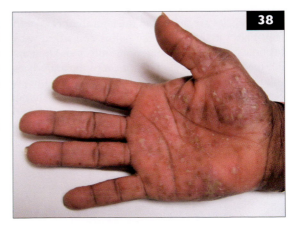

37 i. The ECG, done after similar monitor strip findings, shows prominent U waves suggestive of hypokalemia. Serum potassium was 1.9 mmol/l (1.9 mEq/l). Episodic weakness after heavy exertion is consistent with periodic paralysis. A heterogeneous group of muscle diseases cause periodic paralysis, which is mainly hereditary and divided into hyperkalemic, hypokalemic, and paramyotonic forms. It involves disorders of sodium, potassium, or calcium channels. Hyperthyroidism is associated with hypokalemic periodic paralysis, particularly in Asians. Weakness occurs during rest, often after strenuous exercise or a preceding high carbohydrate meal, although other stresses (e.g. infection) and medications (e.g. insulin) can trigger attacks. Patients awaken with symmetrical or asymmetrical weakness, usually sparing respiratory and facial muscles. Diagnosis is by clinical history and abnormal potassium level. Nerve conduction studies, often enhanced by muscle cooling or exercise, may be diagnostic in unclear cases. Provocative testing with glucose load or IV epinephrine may also help.

ii. Symptomatic hypokalemic periodic paralysis is initially treated by oral potassium replacement, assuming normal renal function. IV potassium is reserved for significant cardiac arrhythmia or respiratory compromise. Continuous cardiac monitoring and serial potassium measurements are mandatory, as is education about potential triggers and evaluation for thyrotoxicosis. Acetazolamide, dichlorphenamide, and, less commonly, potassium-sparing diuretics (e.g. triamterene) have been used in prophylaxis.

38 i. Dyshidrotic eczema, or pompholyx, a recurrent form of vesicular palmoplantar dermatitis of unknown etiology. Many factors trigger episodes, including contact dermatitis to heavy metals (e.g. nickel), dermatophytes, and bacterial infections. Hyperhidrosis is an aggravating factor in 40% of cases. Emotional upset and environmental factors (e.g. seasonal changes) may also cause exacerbations. In mild cases, vesicles are present in the lateral aspects of fingers or, less commonly, toes and feet. Flares may involve the palms and soles, with vesicles and/or bullae that may become pustular and sometimes infected. Diagnosis is usually clinical.

ii. Treatment begins with treatment of the underlying triggers. 10% aluminum acetate solution in a 1:40 dilution or 1:10,000 potassium permanganate compresses will help. Topical corticosteroids are the mainstay of therapy, with systemic corticosteroids reserved for severe episodes. Topical calcineurin inhibitors (e.g. tacrolimus), ultraviolet light plus or minus psoralens, botulinum A toxin injections, and, occasionally, immunosuppressive agents help with refractory cases. Antibiotic therapy and/or drainage of infected bullae may be necessary to control secondary infection.

39 A 32-year-old male presented after being bitten by this spider (39), which he was able to capture.
i. What symptoms is he likely to have?
ii. What other spiders cause significant illness in the world?

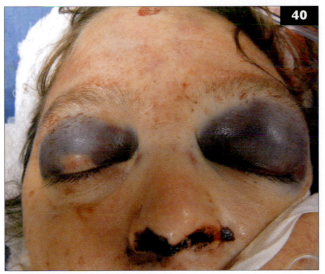

40 A 49-year-old female was the victim of a vicious assault and presented unconscious. No further history was available.
i. What do her eye findings suggest (40)?
ii. How should she be evaluated?

39 i. This is a black widow spider (*Latrodectus* spp.), which causes latrodectism. This 1–2 cm female spider has larger venom glands than the male and can cause serious envenomation. She has a red–orange, hourglass-shaped spot on her ventral abdomen. Many bites do not envenomate. Alpha-latrotoxin is the main toxin, which opens presynaptic calcium channels, with increased neurotransmitter release causing autonomic and neurologic overstimulation. Within 2 hours of envenomation, severe muscle cramps develop, first near the bite and then in the abdomen, back, arms, and thighs. Other symptoms include nausea, vomiting, itching, headache, weakness, dyspnea, and anxiety. There may be hypertension and tachycardia. Death is extremely rare. Treatment includes standard supportive care, judicious use of opiates for pain control, and benzodiazepines for relaxation. Calcium gluconate is no longer recommended. Antivenin is available for those patients severely symptomatic and refractory to the above measures. It resolves symptoms in about 30 minutes, but use must be balanced against allergic risks.

ii. The majority of spiders causing serious bites possess neurotoxin-containing venom. The Australian funnel and mouse spiders, Brazilian wandering spider, and widow spiders work in this manner. Recluse spiders and the six-eyed sand spider produce necrotoxic venom, leading to significant local tissue injury and, occasionally, systemic symptoms.

40 i. These are bilateral periorbital ecchymoses, also known as raccoon or panda eyes. This finding is highly suggestive of basilar skull fracture with resultant blood tracking around the eyes. Other common findings suggestive of basilar skull fracture include mastoid hematoma (Battle sign), bloody otorrhea, hemotympanum, and CSF rhinorrhea. Raccoon eyes may also be seen with direct eye trauma, head or facial surgery, amyloidosis, malignancy, and even vigorous sneezing or coughing.

ii. Supportive care with attention to ABC is appropriate. CT neuroimaging is important to evaluate for basilar skull fracture or other intracranial injury. In this unconscious patient with significant head trauma, the cervical spine should be immobilized and appropriately imaged to rule out associated neck injury. Bedside glucose testing should be done, along with a full evaluation for other trauma.

41 A 27-year-old male presented with new onset of generalized, tonic–clonic seizures. He had a vague psychiatric history and friends stated he has come to believe that drinking a large amount of water would rid him of 'the voices'. He presented unconscious, but not seizing. He was taking unknown psychiatric medications.

i. What laboratory testing should be done promptly?
ii. How should the patient be managed?

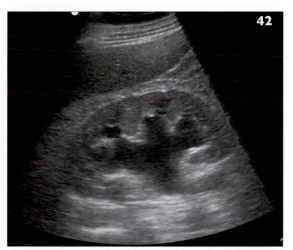

42 A 42-year-old male presented with severe left flank and mid-back pain that radiated down to his left groin. He had a history of renal colic.

i. What does this ultrasound image suggest (42)?
ii. How should the patient be managed?
iii. Is further imaging indicated?

41 i. This patient has psychogenic polydipsia, a disorder seen in mental illness where excessive water consumption leads to dilutional hyponatremia. Severe hyponatremia causes muscle weakness, fatigue, altered mental status, and, occasionally, seizures. Certain psychiatric medications (e.g. phenothiazines) may cause dry mouth, increased thirst, and help create the problem. Serum sodium should be measured promptly and a glucose test done, as hypoglycemia is always part of the differential diagnosis of altered mental status and seizures.

ii. Treatment is dependent on the clinical situation. IV benzodiazepines (e.g. lorazepam) are usually effective at controlling seizures. For coma or intractable seizures with serum sodium significantly below 120 mmol/l (120 mEq/l), rapid, partial correction of hyponatremia with hypertonic saline back to 120 mmol/l improves associated brain edema, usually resolving these problems. This is rarely necessary in psychogenic polydipsia, as patients with normal renal function produce very dilute urine and rapidly correct when they quit drinking. Too rapid correction of severe hyponatremia may contribute to osmotic demyelination syndrome (previously termed central pontine myelinolysis). This may lead to a permanent neurologic deficit, up to and including locked-in syndrome. An evaluation for other contributing etiologies of hyponatremia may be warranted. Psychiatric evaluation and appropriate counseling are often necessary.

42 i. The image shows substantial amounts of hydronephrosis. In a relatively young person with a previous history of renal colic, it defines ureteral obstruction, likely from a stone. Ultrasound is a reasonable screening evaluation for suspected ureteral calculi. It indirectly helps in diagnosis by showing hydronephrosis and hydroureter, but generally does not visualize the stone directly. Although noncontrast spiral CT of the abdomen may give more definitive information, cost and radiation exposure are substantial.

ii. Pain management with NSAIDs and/or narcotics should be initiated promptly. Volume loading with fluids orally or IV will increase urine production and may enhance stone passage. Alpha-1 adrenergic receptor antagonists (e.g. tamsulosin) and calcium channel blockers (e.g. nifedipine) appear to improve spontaneous passage of moderate-sized, distal ureteral stones. Stone size and ureteral position predict the likelihood of expulsion. Most stones 6 mm or less in diameter will pass without urologic intervention, although often taking up to several weeks. Fever or other evidence of urinary tract infection with an obstruction should prompt urgent urologic consultation along with appropriate antibiotic therapy.

iii. In patients with significant risk of renal colic and a suggestive ultrasound, further imaging is probably not necessary.

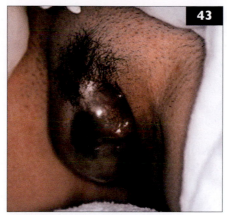

43 An 18-year-old female presented with severe groin pain after vigorous sexual intercourse.
i. What is the clinical problem (**43**)?
ii. How should this patient be evaluated and managed?

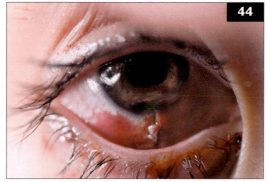

44 A 47-year-old male was involved in a motor vehicle collision as an unrestrained passenger. His only trauma was to the face.
i. What does this photograph suggest (**44**)?
ii. How should the patient be managed?

43 i. This is a large vulvar hematoma, likely due to blunt trauma. Vulvar hematoma is most commonly due to a straddle injury, with the periclitoral vessels crushed against the pubic bone. It is also reported with vaginal delivery, local surgery, and as a postcoital injury. Vulvar hematoma may be associated with coagulopathy. Physical abuse should be considered, and the patient interviewed in a safe, private environment.

ii. Diagnosis of vulvar hematoma is visual, with unilateral painful swelling and ecchymosis of the labial area. Ice therapy is recommended to decrease pain and swelling as well as reduce further bleeding. Significant hematomas may impair voluntary voiding and require a urinary catheter until improved. Pain management with narcotic analgesia is appropriate. Bed rest is generally recommended until improvement, and these simple measures allow most vulvar hematomas to resolve slowly over a few days. Surgical exploration and/or drainage are generally not recommended, except for large hematomas that continue to expand. An alternative therapy for large or expanding vulvar hematomas is transarterial embolization. Coagulopathy work-up should be considered for expanding hematomas and those without a clear etiology.

44 i. In addition to diffuse hemorrhagic chemosis and hyphema, there is a scleral rent with choroid protrusion inferiorly. Globe rupture occurs with any full-thickness injury to the sclera or cornea, representing an ophthalmologic emergency. Blunt trauma usually causes rupture at the insertion of the extraocular muscles, the optic nerve, or the limbus. Penetrating trauma can occur with any object, and foreign body retention is easily missed. Pain, visual loss, and occasionally diplopia are the main complaints in globe rupture, which is often occult. Associated eyelid injury, conjunctival laceration, extensive subconjunctival hemorrhage, corneal or scleral laceration with iris prolapse, irregular pupil, or shallow anterior chamber is suggestive. Measurement of intraocular pressure is contraindicated. The Seidel test uses fluorescein to assess for the presence of aqueous humor streaming, suggesting anterior perforation. CT is the most sensitive imaging modality to detect occult rupture or retained foreign body. MRI is also sensitive, but contraindicated if a ferromagnetic foreign body is suspected.

ii. A suspected globe rupture should be protected with a rigid shield. Broad-spectrum antibiotics should be administered to help prevent infectious endo-phthalmitis. Antiemetics and analgesics are indicated, with appropriate tetanus prophylaxis. Immediate ophthalmologic consultation is necessary, as early surgical management is almost always indicated in globe rupture to maximize vision salvage.

45 A 47-year-old male had left knee arthroscopy the week before he presented with this swollen lower extremity (45a).
i. What does the photograph suggest?
ii. What therapy is indicated?

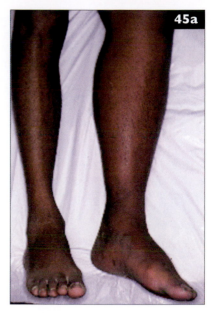

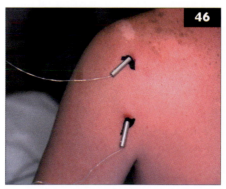

46 A 34-year-old male was brought to the hospital after being shot with a Taser weapon when he became very violent and attacked a police officer. He was initially calm, but became agitated with attempts to remove these barbed projectiles (46).
i. How does this device work, and what are its complications?
ii. How should the patient be managed?

45 i. There is marked, unilateral, lower extremity swelling. Color flow Doppler ultrasound demonstrated a noncompressible proximal left common femoral vein (**45b**, arrows), diagnostic of an intravenous clot and, in this setting, definitive for acute deep venous thrombophlebitis. Because it is proximal to the knee, there is a very high likelihood of embolism to the lungs (>50% without therapy). Vessel wall injury, venous stasis, and hypercoagulable state, the three elements of Virchow's triad,

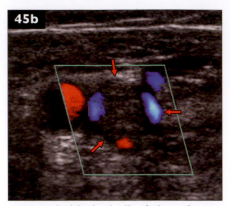

predispose to intravascular clot. This patient probably had all of these factors postoperatively.

ii. Immediate anticoagulation therapy with low molecular weight heparin (e.g. enoxaparin) is proven superior to unfractionated heparin for acute deep venous thrombophlebitis. With severe iliofemoral involvement, catheter-directed thrombolytic therapy and/or mechanical clot removal may be considered. However, no study clearly demonstrates that thrombolysis in typical deep venous thrombophlebitis reduces the incidence of postphlebitic syndrome, the main chronic complication. Vena cava filters should be strongly considered in certain cases, particularly when anticoagulation is either ineffective or contraindicated.

46 i. The Taser is a direct current electrical device used mainly by police forces as an alternative to conventional firearms in dealing with violent or dangerous individuals. The subject is incapacitated by the delivery of rapid pulses of electricity that cause painful, involuntary muscle contractions. Taser use may cause respiratory, cardiovascular, ocular, traumatic, obstetric, and/or biochemical complications. Patients with active illicit substance abuse may be at higher risk of death from Taser weapon use, although controversy exists as studies show proper use of these devices rarely has significant complications. They are clearly safer than bullet injuries from firearms!

ii. The patient should be carefully managed to avoid injury to hospital personnel. A cooperative patient can have the projectile easily removed by stabilizing the surrounding skin while providing inward pressure using one hand and forcefully pulling the single-barb probe with the other hand or something like a pair of pliers. Intradermal lidocaine injection may improve patient comfort during removal.

47 A 24-year-old male awoke with severe pain in his scrotum. He denied recent trauma and had no urinary symptoms. He underwent emergency Doppler ultrasound examination of the scrotum, with this representative image (**47**).

i. Is this the best test to evaluate this patient?

ii. What does the ultrasound image show?

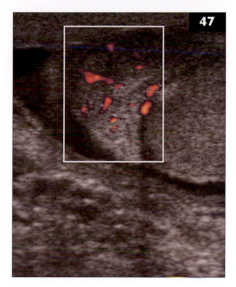

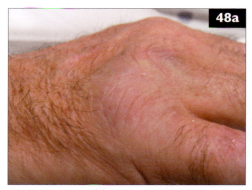

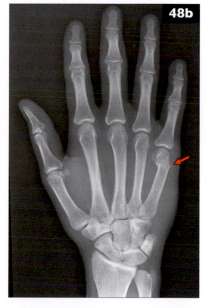

48 A 37-year-old male punched a wall in anger and complained of hand pain (**48a**) A dorsoventral radiograph was obtained (**48b**).

i. What is the likely diagnosis?

ii. How should the condition be managed?

47 i. Acute testicular torsion, a true urologic emergency, must be excluded quickly. The testicle is covered by tunica vaginalis, normally attaching to the posterior scrotal wall. In the bell clapper deformity, there is congenital high or absent tunica vaginalis attachment, allowing testicular rotation around the spermatic cord. Partial torsion occurs if it rotates at least 90°, reducing blood flow. Complete torsion occurs if rotation is 360° or more, with resulting severe ischemia. Testicular torsion happens mostly in males 12–18 years old, but is seen from neonates to elderly. Diagnosis is time urgent, with salvage rates of 90–100% if successful detorsion within 6 hours of pain onset, 20–50% after 12 hours, and <10% if delayed >24 hours. Main physical findings include a tender, elevated testicle with horizontal lie, as well as testicular and scrotal enlargement. Testicular torsion is a clinical diagnosis. If obvious, imaging only delays emergency detorsion, best done bedside or by immediate urologist management. Doppler ultrasound is the optimal imaging modality, with 90–100% sensitivity and specificity. Absent blood flow is the most important finding in testicular torsion, and normal perfusion excludes it. Doppler ultrasound has largely replaced radio-nuclide studies, where decreased testicular uptake correlates with reduced flow.
ii. Increased epididymal blood flow consistent with epididymo-orchitis, an infectious process due to sexually transmitted organisms (*Chlamydia* most common cause if <35 years old) and many gram-negative bacteria. Antibiotic therapy with pain control is appropriate here.

48 i. Boxer's fracture (**48b**, arrow), the common name for a broken fifth (or fourth) finger metacarpal neck, which forms the knuckle. Caused by closed fist impact to a solid object, the metacarpal head tilts volarly and the joint hyperextends. Boxer's fracture presents with swelling, knuckle depression, and pain on range of motion. Laceration over the knuckle may represent a human bite or open fracture, increasing the risk of complications. Rotational deformity is assessed by observing for nail bed rotation, inappropriate medial or ulnar angulation, as well as finger overlap on flexion. Lateral radiographs measure the degree of displacement, with up to 70° often accepted if no significant rotational abnormality.
ii. Fracture reduction is accomplished after a hematoma block or ulnar nerve block. The flexed metacarpal head is directed dorsally to correct volar angulation, and an ulnar gutter splint applied with the metacarpophalangeal joint flexed 90°. Most reductions are relatively unstable. If postreduction lateral radiographs show >30–40° of angulation, there may be some loss of function, with percutaneous pin fixation a consideration. Significant angulation on an anterior–posterior radiograph represents finger malrotation and requires surgical management. Open fractures require surgical irrigation and appropriate antibiotic therapy. Some recommend conservative treatment with taping or bracing that does not restrict movement for closed Boxer's fracture with angulation <70° and no rotational deformity.

49 A 39-year-old male with sickle cell anemia presented with 1 day of increasing headache and neck pain. He had a temperature of 39°C and seemed very ill. BP was 148/80 mmHg (19.7/10.7 kPa) with P 124 bpm.
i. What is the likely diagnosis, and how should it be confirmed?
ii. What treatment is indicated?

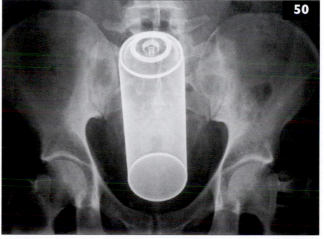

50 A 39-year-old male presented with rectal bleeding and stated that someone may have put something 'up there' while he was intoxicated.
i. Any guess what the object is (50)?
ii. How should the patient be managed?

49 i. Sickle cell anemia is associated with functional asplenia and an immuno-compromised state. These patients are at risk for serious infection, particularly by encapsulated organisms. Although various types of infection are possible here, an immediate concern is meningitis. Immunosuppressed patients have reduced inflammatory response to infection, including meningeal signs. Appropriate testing includes CBC as well as cultures of blood and urine. Lumbar puncture should be performed immediately. Although CT has been suggested in this clinical situation to exclude an intracranial mass lesion, it is unnecessary in the absence of lateralizing neurologic signs or altered mental status, and may delay appropriate diagnosis as well as therapy.

ii. Antipyretics and IV fluids should be initiated. Immediate broad-spectrum antibiotic therapy is appropriate, often with an extended-spectrum penicillin or cephalosporin along with vancomycin (for antimicrobial-resistant gram-positive cocci). IV dexamethasone should be initiated at once, ideally before antibiotics, and repeated dosing has been shown to reduce mortality in bacterial meningitis. These interventions should begin even before lumbar puncture if it cannot be accomplished immediately. Supportive therapy is important.

50 i. A very large spray can! Rectal foreign bodies come in an amazing variety of sizes and shapes, generally inserted through the anus. The history is often unreliable. Although most are inserted as part of erotic activity, a high index of suspicion for sexual violence must be maintained. Occasionally, rectal foreign bodies are inserted to hide the object (e.g. weapons), and some are initially swallowed and become impacted in the rectum (e.g. sunflower seeds). Objects below the sacral curve and rectosigmoid junction are generally easily visualized and removed, while higher lying objects are often unreachable through the anus. Often, multiple attempts at self-removal have occurred. There may be mucosal injury with edema, bleeding, or even frank perforation.

ii. An appropriate caring and respectful attitude is essential. Radiography will help identify the object and reveal evidence of perforation (e.g. free air). A sedated evaluation is important, as is ingenuity with use of balloon devices, gynecologic forceps, and anal dilators for removal. Except in simple cases, surgical consultation is important, as some require laparotomy for removal. Remember to do no harm, which may occur with bowel injury due to instrumentation or discharge of some devices (e.g. rectal gun).

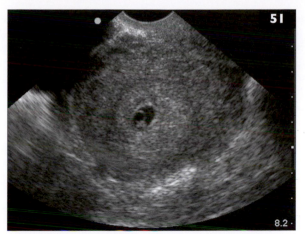

51 An 18-year-old female presented with lower abdominal pain and minor vaginal bleeding.
i. What does this transvaginal ultrasound image show (51)?
ii. Can the patient be reassured?

52 A 37-year-old male presented with severe, crampy, right flank pain radiating into his groin, along with nausea and vomiting. He had gross hematuria.
i. What is the likely diagnosis?
ii. How would you confirm the diagnosis?

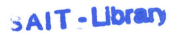

51 i. An intrauterine pregnancy with a gestational sac, yolk sac, and embryo. Using transvaginal ultrasonography, a gestational sac is usually visible 4.5 weeks after the last day of the previous menstrual period, a yolk sac at about 5 weeks, and an embryo at 5.5 weeks. Fetal heart activity is usually apparent when the embryo is 5 mm or more in size, usually around 6 weeks gestational age. Similar trans-abdominal ultrasound findings are each delayed by about a week, respectively.

ii. The main causes of first-trimester vaginal bleeding include implantation bleeding, ectopic pregnancy, spontaneous abortion, perineal infections, and diseases involving the female reproductive tract. This patient has an intrauterine pregnancy at 5.5–6 weeks and her ultrasound may or may not show fetal heart activity. If fetal heart activity is detected, the likelihood of continued pregnancy is over 95%. This information allows appropriate reassurance and discharge. It is unclear if bed rest has any true effect in threatened abortion, but limited physical activity until obstetric follow-up seems sensible. Prescribe prenatal vitamins.

52 i. Acute flank pain has a small differential diagnosis including mainly musculo-skeletal problems and renal issues, particularly pyelonephritis and renal colic. Crampy intermittent pain is suggestive of a hollow viscus source such as renal colic. Usually this pain with hematuria is due to renal colic. However, hematuria is absent in 25–30% of patients on initial urinalysis who prove to have ureteral stones. Other etiologies of acute flank or back pain must be considered (especially ruptured abdominal aortic aneurysm in older patients). Physical examination may be helpful for exclusion, as renal colic usually presents with a relatively benign abdomen and back.

ii. Abdominal radiography may reveal stones, but has high false-negative rates. Ultrasound is suggestive in most cases, showing hydronephrosis and hydroureter, but may miss up to 15–20% of ureteral stones, as some are minimally obstructing. IV pyelography is very sensitive, showing a delayed nephrogram along with evidence of ureteral obstruction, but has contrast issues. Noncontrasted CT has become the diagnostic modality of choice in many centers, as it has high sensitivity and specificity, may recognize other etiologies, but requires no IV contrast (52).

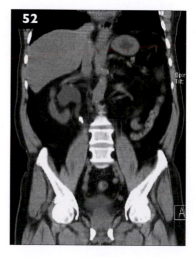

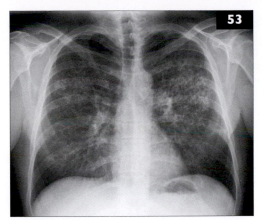

53 A 45-year-old male presented with increasing shortness of breath over the past 5 days. He had a history of HIV and had been noncompliant with his HAART therapy. A recent CD4 count was 55 cells/µl. He had a previous severe rash with trimethoprim-sulfamethoxazole.
i. What does this chest radiograph suggest (53)?
ii. How should it be treated?

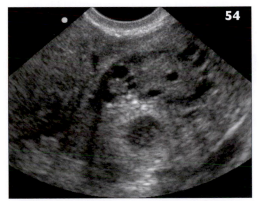

54 A 27-year-old female presented with mild lower abdominal pain. She did not believe she could be pregnant, but was unsure about timing of her last menstrual period. She had normal vital signs and minimal tenderness in her lower abdomen.
i. What does this ultrasound show (54)?
ii. Are there new considerations in the management of this patient?

53 i. Extensive bilateral perihilar pneumonitis, which in this clinical setting is probably due to *Pneumocystis jirovecii*, a yeast-like fungus that only infects humans. Found in lungs of most healthy people, it becomes an opportunistic infection in the immunocompromised host, including those with HIV and a CD4 count under about 200 cells/µl, malignancy, or on immunosuppressive medications (e.g. chemotherapy). *Pneumocystis* pneumonia presents with fever, nonproductive cough, and shortness of breath developing over days to weeks. Diagnosis is usually made by recognition of characteristic 'bat-wing' infiltrates on the chest radiograph. Significant hypoxia is common. Sputum can be stained (e.g. with silver stain) to show typical cysts. Rarely, *Pneumocystis* pneumonia is diagnosed by broncho-alveolar lavage or lung biopsy.

ii. The most common treatment is trimethoprim–sulfamethoxazole, which is also used in AIDS patients with a low CD4 count to suppress this infectious agent. This patient is allergic to that antibiotic. Other medications used for *Pneumocystis* pneumonia, either alone or in combination, include clindamycin, pentamidine, dapsone, atovaquone, primaquine, trimetrexate, and investigational agents. Infectious disease specialists should be consulted in complex cases. Hypoxia is treated with supplemental oxygen. Corticosteroids are shown to increase survival with significant hypoxia (pO_2 <70 mmHg [9.3 kPa]).

54 i. The transvaginal ultrasound image reveals a thick-walled, fluid-filled structure adjacent to the ovary that appears to have an embryo in it. It did, with a heartbeat. Further ultrasound images showed no evidence of intra-abdominal hemorrhage.

ii. Many women with uncomplicated ectopic pregnancy are now treated with methotrexate rather than conventional surgery. The patient must be hemo-dynamically stable without evidence of active bleeding or hemoperitoneum. The ectopic mass should be less than 3.5 cm in greatest dimension by ultrasound. Those with beta-hCG levels <3,000 IU/l (optimally <1,500 IU/l) are usual candidates for methotrexate. Patients must be reliable, compliant, available for follow-up, and without contraindications to methotrexate. A single dose of methotrexate, with repeat dosing based on response, is highly successful and may conserve reproductive function. Patients must be warned to return promptly if signs of substantial intra-abdominal bleeding develop.

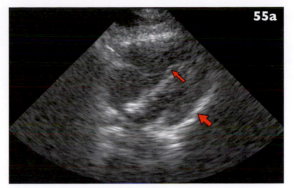

55 A previously healthy 37-year-old female presented with acute severe dyspnea. She was a couple of weeks postpartum. BP was 94/60 mmHg (12.5/8.0 kPa), P 140 bpm, RR 36/min, and P_{ox} 96% on room air.
i. What does this cardiac ultrasound suggest (55a)?
ii. What intervention is indicated?

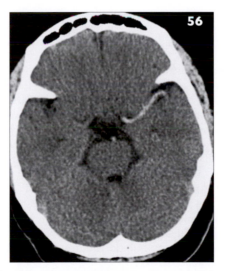

56 A 59-year-old male with a history of hypertension and diabetes mellitus presented with acute right-sided weakness and inability to speak, which began about 2.5 hours prior to arrival. BP was 210/120 mmHg (28.0/16.0 kPa) with P 68 bpm.
i. What does this CT image suggest (56)?
ii. How should the patient be managed?

55 i. The normal right ventricular (RV) (55a, thin arrow) to left ventricular (LV) (55a, thick arrow) diameter ratio is <0.7. In this case, it is near 1, suggesting RV dilatation. In this clinical setting, that is highly suggestive of acute pulmonary embolism with significant right-sided hemodynamic obstruction.

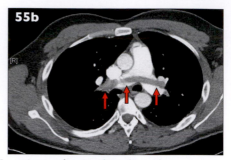

ii. Although some clinicians may want confirmation of acute pulmonary emboli by immediate contrasted pulmonary CT angiography, in this clinical scenario a hemodynamically significant pulmonary embolism is highly likely. CT revealed this large venous-shaped clot (55b, arrows). Thrombolytic therapy (e.g. tissue plasminogen activator) is recommended in pulmonary embolism with hemodynamic instability, right-sided heart strain, or high-risk patients with poor cardiopulmonary reserve. However, no randomized clinical trials have proven conclusively that thrombolytics are superior to anticoagulation with heparin in this setting. Interventional radiologic techniques to fragment and extract the clot are used in specialized centers and, along with thoracic surgery for clot removal, may be life saving.

56 i. The clinical situation suggests acute left hemispheric stroke with symptom onset approaching the most accepted 3-hour time limit for thrombolytic therapy. CT reveals a hyperdense left middle cerebral artery sign, sometimes seen with acute thrombus formation. It is indicative of an impending large infarct with poor prognosis, but may be mimicked by atherosclerotic changes.

ii. The hyperdense middle cerebral artery sign is not in itself a contraindication to thrombolytic therapy in acute stroke. However, this patient is unlikely to have complete clinical evaluation, brain CT with interpretation, and infusion of thrombolytic therapy in the remaining 30 minutes. Although recent research suggests some benefit in extending the thrombolytic treatment window in acute nonhemorrhagic stroke to 4.5 hours, this industry-sponsored study has had some criticism. In addition, the patient has a BP well above limits recognized as contraindications to thrombolytic therapy in stroke (SBP >185 mmHg [24.7 kPa] or DBP >110 mmHg [14.7 kPa] at infusion time). The net therapeutic benefit of thrombolytic therapy in acute stroke remains somewhat controversial. Many patients present late, have unclear time of symptom onset, have stroke mimics, or have contraindications to thrombolytic therapy. We remain in our infancy in improving outcomes in acute stroke.

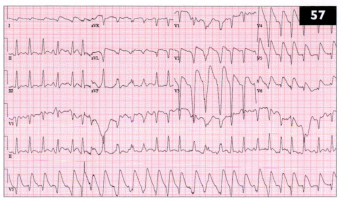

57 A 63-year-old patient had a history of hypertension and ongoing cocaine abuse. He presented with 1 hour of severe chest pain, shortness of breath, palpitations, diaphoresis, and this ECG (57).
i. What does the ECG reveal?
ii. What treatment is indicated?

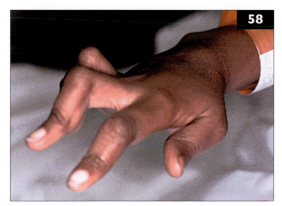

58 A 35-year-old female had an acute exacerbation of chronic arthritis in many of her joints. She was not on any medications.
i. What does this photograph suggest is the cause of the arthritis (58)?
ii. What treatments are appropriate?

57 i. The ECG is very interesting and requires a systematic analysis. There is a rapid irregular rhythm, which excludes ventricular tachycardia since that has a consistently regular pattern. Looking at the lead II rhythm strip, it is actually possible to see at least three different P wave shapes, so this is multifocal atrial tachycardia with a ventricular rate of approximately 156 bpm. There is marked ST segment elevation with q waves in leads V_1 to V_6, consistent with acute anterolateral STEMI. There are also occasional wide-complex beats of unclear etiology.

ii. This patient should undergo immediate percutaneous coronary intervention. Thrombolytic therapy is relatively contraindicated, as cocaine-induced vasospasm rather than intracoronary thrombosis may be etiologic of these ECG findings. Beta-blockers are also contraindicated, as they may increase vasospasm by decreasing beta-2 adrenergic receptor-induced vasodilation. Oxygen, aspirin, enoxaparin, IV fluid boluses, nitrates, and benzodiazepines are all reasonable here. In particular, benzodiazepines may reduce systemic catecholamines by central GABA receptor stimulation.

58 i. The patient has evidence of severe rheumatoid arthritis (RA), an autoimmune disease that causes chronic inflammation in many joints and surrounding tissues. It affects millions of patients worldwide and is three times more common in women. RA is a systemic illness that can involve any joint, but the upper and lower extremities are most commonly affected. The joints are erythematous and swollen, with pain on range of motion. This case shows chronic changes in the fingers (i.e. contractures, Boutonnière deformities) with wrist and finger joint inflammation. Other manifestations of RA include spine involvement with potential instability as well as rheumatoid vasculitis, which may involve the heart, lungs, nervous system, and other organs.

ii. Standard therapy for RA includes NSAIDs (e.g. diclofenac). Intermittent therapy with corticosteroids (e.g. prednisone) may help control flares, and they are frequently used in low doses for chronic inflammation control. Disease-modifying antirheumatic drugs are the current standard of care for severe RA, as in this case, with methotrexate most commonly used. Antimalarials (e.g. hydroxychloroquine), specific white cell modulators (e.g. rituximab), and tumor necrosis factor alpha inhibitors (e.g. infliximab) are other classes of medications used selectively after rheumatologist evaluation.

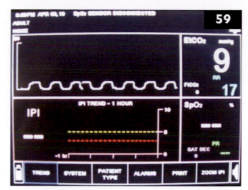

59 A 21-year-old male presented with altered mental status and obvious severe dyspnea. No history was available. BP was 130/80 mmHg (17.3/10.7 kPa) with P 124 bpm, RR 18/min, and T 35.3°C.
i. What does his capnography suggest (59)?
ii. What bedside test is important here?

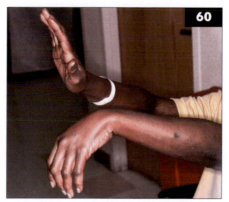

60 A 33-year-old male had a history of alcohol abuse and presented with left wrist weakness. On examination he had normal left bicep, tricep, and wrist flexor strength. The photograph shows what happened when he attempted to extend his left wrist (60).
i. What does this finding suggest?
ii. Can this patient's problem be fixed in time for a date (!) tonight?

59 i. Capnography reveals end-tidal CO_2 of 9 mmHg (1.2 kPa), suggesting near-maximal hyperventilation, likely in response to severe metabolic acidosis.

ii. The patient has respiratory compensation for severe metabolic acidosis, and significant hypothermia. Diabetic ketoacidosis, a prime consideration, is due to absolute or relative insulin deficiency with increased levels of counter-regulatory hormones (glucagon, cortisol, catecholamines, growth hormone). In both hypoglycemia and diabetic ketoacidosis, glucose cannot enter cells, so metabolism is decreased and hypothermia common. Glucose should be promptly measured (here was 70 mmol/l [1,262 mg/dl]); laboratory studies confirmed diabetic ketoacidosis: serum acetone positive at 1:64 dilution, Na 120 mmol/l (120 mEq/l), K 6.2 mmol/l (6.2 mEq/l), Cl 89 mmol/l (89 mEq/l), CO_2 6 mmol/l (6 mEq/l), and Cr 124 µmol/l (1.4 mg/dl). Corrected sodium level is about 140 mmol/l (add 1.6 mmol/l [1.6 mEq/l] for each 5.6 mmol/l [100 mg/dl] of glucose above 5.6 mmol/l [100 mg/dl]). The patient needs crystalloid infusion (20 ml/kg a good start), insulin IV at about 0.1 units/kg/hour, and early potassium replacement when levels begin to drop (total body potassium depletion masked by severe acidosis). Evaluate for and manage infection, which commonly triggers diabetic ketoacidosis. Other precipitating causes include noncompliance with insulin therapy and intercurrent illnesses (e.g. myocardial infarction, pancreatitis, trauma, recent surgery, and other stressors).

60 i. A radial nerve injury due to prolonged compression of the inside arm against a hard object, commonly called 'Saturday night palsy'. Most often, it occurs when a patient falls asleep with his arm thrown over a chair. It may be secondary to other compressive mechanisms, such as a direct blow. Alcohol intoxication often contributes. This is a neuropraxia, where there is internal biochemical damage to the nerve, but no break in the internal axon (axonotmesis) or nerve itself (neurotmesis). Paralysis to wrist and finger extensors occurs, with some related sensory deficits.

ii. Weakness may resolve within hours, but on average it takes up to 6–8 weeks for recovery of normal strength. No definitive therapy for this radial nerve neuropraxia exists. Physical therapy to preserve range of motion and counseling about avoiding further nerve compression are appropriate. Time is the only cure for this problem. Hopefully, his date will understand.

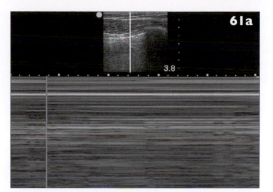

61 A 27-year-old female presented with acute right chest pain and shortness of breath after involvement in a motor vehicle collision.
i. What does this M-mode ultrasound image suggest (**61a**)?
ii. What treatment is indicated?

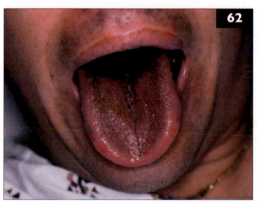

62 A 27-year-old male presented with recent severe diarrhea and complained that he was lightheaded and weak.
i. What does this photograph suggest (**62**)?
ii. Is any treatment necessary?

61 i. Ultrasound is useful in evaluation for suspected pneumothorax. Normally, a high-resolution linear ultrasound probe can recognize movement of the visceral pleura and underlying lung in relation to the fixed parietal pleura ('lung sliding'). Also, changes in acoustic impedance at the pleura–lung interface result in horizontal artifacts visible as a series of echogenic parallel lines equidistant from one another below the pleural line.

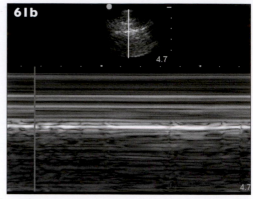

Finally, vertically oriented comet tail artifacts are seen at the pleural interface with normal lung. Presence of lung sliding with comet tail artifacts has a near 100% negative predictive value for pneumothorax at that level. Another sign ('lung point') occurs in pneumothorax, where a precisely placed probe shows lung sliding along with comet tails in inspiration, which disappears on expiration. In M-mode, normal lung has smooth lines above the pleural line, but the image is grainy below ('seashore sign') (**61b**). The M-mode ultrasound (**61a**) shows a 'stratosphere sign', with smooth lines below the pleural line ('A lines') consistent with pneumothorax.
ii. Bedside ultrasound alone cannot quantitate pneumothorax size and may miss small ones. If clinically indicated, pleural decompression is the treatment of choice for significant pneumothorax.

62 i. The black tongue results from staining with bismuth sulfide. Sulfur, found in saliva, combines with bismuth subsalicylate (in Pepto Bismol, an antidiarrheal drug) to produce this finding. Black licorice, tobacco, beetroot, and certain red wines or black teas may cause similar staining. Other medications, including some antacids, analgesics, antidepressants, antihypertensives, antimicrobials, and chemotherapeutic agents, can lead to an acquired macular lingual pigmentation.
ii. No treatment is necessary for this tongue staining, just reassurance, as it will resolve over a few days. However, it may be useful to evaluate the patients's electrolytes and hydration status and treat as necessary. Also, a rectal examination with occult blood testing should be performed to exclude significant gastrointestinal bleed. Antispasmodics may be useful to reduce diarrhea.

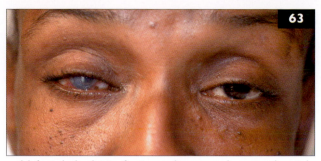

63 A 38-year-old female had Marfan's syndrome and received a right eye corneal transplant 2 years ago. She had noted increased pain and redness in that eye over the past 2 weeks, with decreased visual acuity (63).
i. What do you think is going on?
ii. Can the corneal transplant be salvaged?

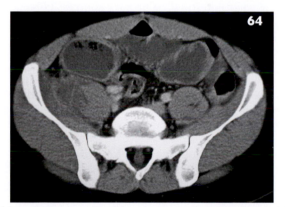

64 A 23-year-old male presented with a history of regional enteritis, severe mid-abdominal pain over the past 24 hours, and vomiting, but no diarrhea. On examination, he had mild diffuse abdominal tenderness with a small wound draining purulent fluid at the right iliac crest.
i. What is the diagnosis (CT scan, 64), and what caused it?
ii. How is the condition treated?

63 i. There is evidence of corneal transplant rejection, which occurs in more than one-third of keratoplasty (corneal transplant) patients by 5 years. It occurs by an immunologic mechanism and is the most common cause of corneal graft failure in the late postoperative period. Any of the three corneal layers (epithelium, stroma, endothelium) can be rejected separately, but many patients demonstrate a combined layer rejection. Although corneal graft rejection may be asymptomatic, eye redness, pain, irritation, photophobia, and decreased visual acuity are common complaints. Corneal clouding, vascularization, and sometimes fluorescein uptake may be seen on examination. Distinguishing the fine details of corneal transplant rejection are complicated and best left to the ophthalmologist.

ii. Aggressive topical corticosteroids are the mainstay of treatment of corneal transplant rejection. Systemic or subconjunctival corticosteroids may be given in difficult cases, and other immunosuppressive agents have been used. Intraocular pressure should be monitored closely. This cornea is unlikely to be salvaged.

64 i. A right-sided iliopsoas abscess, an unusual cause of abdominal pain. About 20% are primary, with 80% due to contiguous spread from infections in the spinal, gastrointestinal, or urinary tract. *Staphylococcus aureus* is usually cultured from primary iliopsoas abscesses and those from bone. *Escherichia coli* is the common bacterial cause for gastrointestinal or urinary sources. Polymicrobial infections occur in 20%. Iliopsoas abscesses occur more frequently in immunocompromised hosts, particularly AIDS, diabetes mellitus, and IV drug users. It presents with fever and complaints of back or abdominal pain. Examination shows back or abdominal tenderness, sometimes with a local mass or draining fistulae, as in this case. Iliopsoas abscesses may demonstrate a positive psoas sign, elicited by the patient lying on the side away from the suspected problem, with abdominal pain elicited when the involved side extremity is extended. Leukocytosis is common and blood cultures may grow the offending organism, as may urine. Imaging is best accomplished with CT or MRI.

ii. Treatment mainly involves appropriate antibiotics and surgical drainage. Initial antibiotics should cover *S. aureus* and enteric bacteria, later tailored by culture results from abscess fluid, blood, or urine. Drainage is essential, with surgical management probably superior to percutaneous drainage.

65 A 47-year-old male construction worker thought he had hurt his shoulder 1 month ago, but did not recall specific trauma. He smoked cigarettes and drank large amounts of alcohol daily. Recently, he had been losing weight with increased cough.

i. What does the chest radiograph suggest (65a)?

ii. How should he be evaluated and managed?

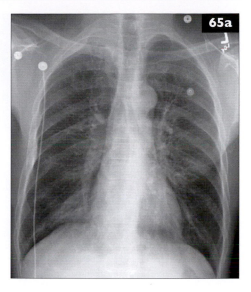

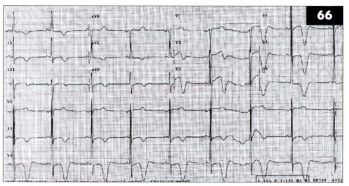

66 A 51-year-old male had a history of hypertension and alcoholism. He was found unconscious at home. BP was 224/90 mmHg (29.9/12.0 kPa), with P 50 bpm, irregular RR 12/min, and T 37.4°C. He had dilated, unreactive pupils and did not move with verbal or mechanical stimulation.

i. What does this ECG suggest (66)?

ii. What evaluation is necessary?

65 i. A Pancoast tumor, or superior sulcus tumor (65b, arrow), a pulmonary neoplasm that typically invades local nerves (brachial plexus, vagus, recurrent laryngeal, phrenic, sympathetic ganglion), blood vessels (subclavian and branchiocephalic), bones (ribs, vertebral bodies), and lung. These are almost always non-small cell lung cancers. They typically present with ipsilateral shoulder and upper extremity pain as well as late weakness. Other complaints include Horner's syndrome (ptosis, miosis, and anhidrosis), and those symptoms related to invasion of the chest wall or vertebral column.

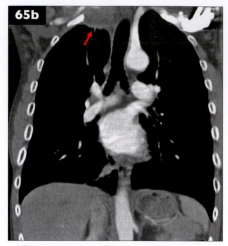

ii. Although previously considered incurable, superior sulcus tumors have an improving prognosis due to a multidisciplinary approach. Diagnosis is usually made histologically by transthoracic needle biopsy. CT, MRI, and/or bone scanning are necessary to evaluate for metastatic disease (65b). Surgical resection is recommended if there are no distant metastases, no extensive mediastinal adenopathy, and if cardiopulmonary status allows. Radiation therapy and chemotherapy prolong survival in unresectable tumors.

66 i. The ECG shows sinus bradycardia with ventricular rate about 50 bpm and very deep T wave inversions in almost every lead. It is unlikely these diffuse T wave inversions are due to myocardial ischemia or pericarditis. Repolarization and ischemic-like ECG changes are frequently observed during the acute phase of stroke, as are prominent U waves and QT interval prolongation. They are particularly common in patients with subarachnoid and intracerebral hemorrhage. Here, the deep, bizarre T wave inversions are termed 'cerebral', 'neurogenic', or 'giant' T waves. Sinus bradycardia is also common. The Cushing's triad, which includes systolic hypertension, irregular respirations, and bradycardia, comprises the Cushing reflex. This is seen in the terminal stages of increased intracranial pressure.
ii. This patient needs definitive airway management, probably by endotracheal intubation after careful, rapid sequence induction. A bedside glucose is important. Early brain CT imaging will define the neurologic injury and prognosis. Here, it showed a large intracerebral hemorrhage with evidence of brain herniation.

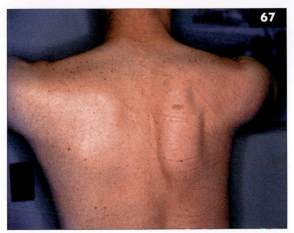

67 A 24-year-old male presented a few days after a painful fall while playing basketball. He complained of pain and difficulty raising his right arm above his shoulder.
i. What is this problem (**67**)?
ii. How is it managed?

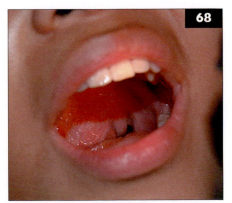

68 A 19-year-old female had a severe sore throat for 2–3 days, fever to 38.7°C, and these findings on clinical examination (**68**).
i. What does the photograph suggest?
ii. How should she be managed?

67 i. A right-sided medial winging of the scapula, made more visible by having the patient push against a wall. In this winged scapula, the medial scapula is not held tight against the back, usually due to serratus anterior muscle dysfunction from injury to the long thoracic nerve. The serratus anterior muscle attaches to the medial anterior aspect of the scapula and anchors it, as well as assisting in scapular rotation when the arm is raised. Lateral winging may be seen with trapezius dysfunction due to accessory nerve injury, which may have a delayed presentation because the trapezius has to stretch for the deformity to be visible. Osseous and soft tissue causes also occur. Winged scapula is relatively rare and is usually due to traumatic compression of the long thoracic or accessory nerve. It has been reported with poor positioning during long operations. Besides cosmetic issues, winged scapula can cause functional shoulder problems. The diagnosis is generally clinical, but CT and electromyelography may better define the problem.

ii. Conservative therapy for up to 2 years has allowed recovery in many cases. Surgical nerve repair, muscle transfer procedures, and even scapulothoracic fusion have been described.

68 i. Exudative pharyngitis with bilateral tonsillar enlargement and leftward uvular deviation suggests right peritonsillar abscess complicating acute tonsillitis. A mixed aerobic and anaerobic bacterial abscess develops between the palatine tonsil and its capsule. Peritonsillar abscess presents with fever and an increasingly sore throat, which can progress to severe dysphagia with muffled voice. Severe tonsillar swelling with erythema is present, along with uvular deviation away from the abscess. Laboratory testing is rarely helpful. Intraoral ultrasound using an intracavitary probe is highly sensitive. CT (rarely needed) may show a hypodense fluid collection with surrounding hyperemia.

ii. In experienced hands, needle aspiration is both diagnostic and therapeutic. Use a 16 or 18 gauge needle with syringe to aspirate the abscess after local anesthesia (e.g. lidocaine with epinephrine). A needle guard (cut 1 cm off needle cover tip) helps prevent carotid artery puncture. Since most abscesses are in the superior pole, aspirate here first. If no purulent fluid is returned, try the middle and finally the inferior pole. Peritonsillar abscesses are rarely significantly loculated. A scalpel may be used in selected cases. Suction must be available. Penicillin, with or without metronidazole (to enhance anaerobic coverage), is recommended, with clindamycin if penicillin allergy. A long-acting corticosteroid (e.g. dexamethasone) may be useful. Otolaryngology follow-up is appropriate, with prompt consultation in difficult cases or if uncomfortable with drainage techniques. Tonsillectomy is sometimes appropriate, particularly for recurrent peritonsillar abscess.

69 A 25-year-old female presented with severe agitation, BP of 180/110 mmHg (24.0/14.7 kPa), P 184 bpm, T 41.2°C, and RR 44/min. She was flushed, but not sweating. Her friend said she drank some homemade tea to 'get high'. She brought a flower from which the tea was made.

i. What is this flower (**69**), and does it relate to this clinical picture?

ii. What management is suggested?

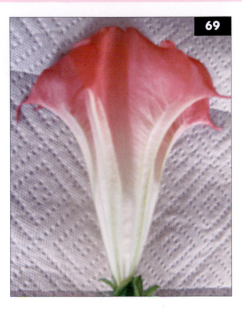

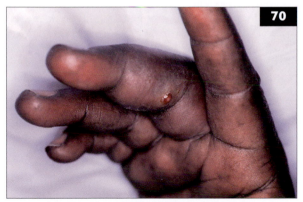

70 A 34-year-old male presented after a minor puncture wound to his finger at work 4 days ago. He cannot straighten his finger fully, and pain is greatly increased by trying to extend it (**70**).

i. What do you have to think about here?

ii. How should he be treated?

69 i. The patient has anticholinergic toxicity. Classic clinical findings include tachycardia, hypertension, hyperthermia, flushing, dry skin, as well as mental status changes with agitation and seizures. These symptoms, as well as mydriasis, ileus, and urinary retention, are due to decreased cholinergic autonomic tone. The mneumonic 'blind as a bat, dry as a bone, red as a beet, mad as a hatter, and hot as a hare' helps recognize anticholinergic toxicity. Anticholinergic toxidrome is distinguished from sympathomimetic overdose by absence of sweating. Common causes include antihistamines (e.g. diphenhydramine), often in sleep aid and cold preparations, tricyclic antidepressants (e.g. amitriptyline), and many plants (e.g. Angel's trumpet, or *Brugmansia*, seen here) containing various belladonna alkaloids. **ii.** Supportive therapy is usually sufficient. Oral decontamination is rarely accomplished safely due to altered mental status. Physostigmine, a reversible cholinesterase inhibitor, should only be used in severe cholinergic poisoning unresponsive to supportive measures, intractable seizures not controlled by benzodiazepines, tachyarrhythmias with hemodynamic compromise, or extreme agitation. Physostigmine may induce a life-threatening cholinergic crisis (seizures, asystole, and/or respiratory depression) and should be avoided in patients using tricyclic antidepressants, type Ia antiarrhythmics (e.g. procainamide), or cocaine. Benzodiazepines (e.g. lorazepam) are useful in less severe cases and reasonably effective.

70 i. Finger injuries are common and may cause secondary infection with serious consequences. In this case there is obvious erythema, with fusiform finger swelling as well as visible subcutaneous purulent fluid. Infection can involve tendon, muscle, joint, or bone. Inability to extend the finger suggests flexor tenosynovitis, which involves tendon sheaths and sometimes spreads rapidly to deep spaces of the hand and beyond. Kanaval's signs for flexor tenosynovitis are: (1) finger held in slight flexion; (2) fusiform swelling; (3) pain with passive finger extension; and (4) tenderness along the flexor tendon sheath. Not surprisingly, *Staphylococcus aureus* is the main organism, but many are mixed infections. Atypical organisms are associated with unusual injuries (e.g. *Pasteurella multocida* with cat bites). Associated joint infections and foreign bodies should also be considered.
ii. Perform radiography to exclude foreign body, and culture fluid obtained by surgical drainage. For early infection (not this case!), IV antibiotics to cover likely organisms are sometimes adequate. Immunocompromised patients and those with foreign body, severe infection, or failure to improve rapidly with antibiotics require surgical drainage. These infections are often more complex than initially recognized, and an experienced hand or orthopedic surgeon should be consulted for definitive operative management.

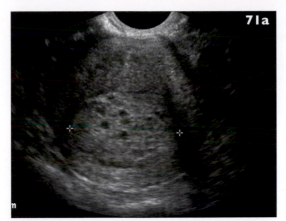

71 An 18-year-old female presented with vaginal bleeding along with nausea and vomiting over the past 5–6 weeks. She was sexually active and her pregnancy test was positive.
i. What does this ultrasound image suggest (71a)?
ii. How should she be treated?

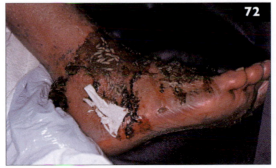

72 A 59-year-old patient with a history of alcoholism presented with this wound (72).
i. What do you see?
ii. Is there any therapeutic benefit?

71 i. The honeycomb appearance of this large amount of intrauterine tissue is very suggestive of molar pregnancy (also called a hydatidiform mole). This is a type of gestational trophoblastic disease more common in very young and older mothers. It may be complete (no normal fetal tissue) or incomplete (mixed fetal and trophoblastic tissue). Hydatidiform moles are benign, occurring in about 1 in 1,000 pregnancies, and more

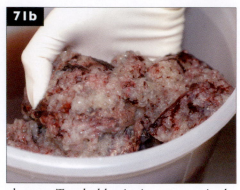

71b

common in women of African or Asian descent. Trophoblastic tissue grows in the placenta as grape-like vesicles up to 1 centimeter in diameter (71b). On ultrasound, this appears like a honeycomb or snowstorm in the uterine cavity, without visible fetal tissue. Molar pregnancies usually present in the third to fifth month with painless vaginal bleeding, uterus often large for dates, frequent vomiting, and possibly elevated BP. Very high levels of beta-hCG are present. Hydatidiform moles may transform to malignant choriocarcinoma.

ii. Immediate gynecologic consultation is indicated. Molar pregnancies should undergo surgical curettage or suction evacuation as soon as possible to lower choriocarcinoma risk. Serial beta-hCG levels are measured until undetectable to confirm resolution. Invasive or metastatic trophoblastic disease may require chemotherapy. Chance of recurrence with subsequent pregnancy is about 1%.

72 i. This right foot and ankle has extensive cellulitis, some ruptured bullae, and a lot of eschar. There are also a large number of maggots in the wound along with a small amount of toilet paper.

ii. Maggots have been used for centuries in the treatment of wounds and infected bone. They aggressively consume necrotic material, but do not attack healthy tissue. Prior to the introduction of antibiotics, maggots were used successfully to treat chronic or infected wounds as well as mastoiditis, chronic empyema, osteomyelitis, burns, and abscesses. Maggot therapy was reintroduced about 20 years ago and has been recently used in at least 20 countries to debride chronic wounds. It is doubtful this patient knew much about the literature concerning maggot therapy.

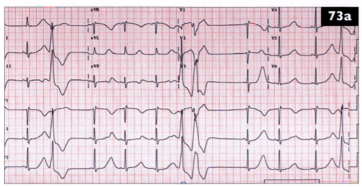

73 A 39-year-old male presented with 1 day of recurrent, pleuritic chest pain along with multiple episodes of vomiting and diarrhea. He had a history of schizophrenia, but did not recall the names of his psychiatric medications, which, surprisingly, he took. He admitted to heavy alcohol, tobacco, and crack cocaine use. He passed out and fell yesterday.
i. What does this ECG show, and what are likely causes (73a)?
ii. What common arrhythmia is associated with this ECG, and how is it treated?

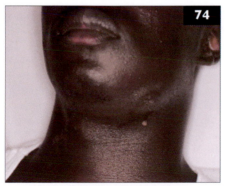

74 A 23-year-old male had several days of dental pain and arrived with facial swelling along with drainage from his left jaw area.
i. What is going on here (74)?
ii. What treatment is indicated?

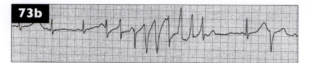

73 i. NSR at about 70 bpm, frequent premature ventricular contractions, and prolonged QT interval. QT interval, measured from start of QRS complex to end of T wave, represents duration of ventricular activation and recovery. Rate correction is standard, with $QT_{corrected} = QT_{measured}$/square root of RR interval (here 0.68; normal $QT_{corrected} = 0.44 \pm 0.04$ seconds). Prolonged QT interval has many causes, particularly certain electrolyte depletions (low K, Mg or Ca). Medications prolonging QT interval include type Ia and III antiarrhythmics, macrolide or quinolone antibiotics, as well as many antihistamines and antipsychotics. Consider congenital prolonged QT syndromes, myocarditis, subarachnoid hemorrhage, and other rare causes. This patient had low potassium (3.1 mmol/l [3.1 mEq/l]) and magnesium (0.6 mmol/l [1.5 mg/dl]) from alcohol abuse along with gastrointestinal losses. His antipsychotic medications included QT interval prolonging quetiapine and sertraline. Cocaine also acts like a type Ia antiarrhythmic to lengthen the QT interval.

ii. Torsade de pointes (**73b**), an unstable type of polymorphic ventricular tachy-cardia particularly associated with prolonged QT interval. It can be prevented by withdrawing offending agent(s), replacing potassium and/or magnesium, temporary overdrive cardiac pacing, or, rarely, IV isoproterenol. Defibrillation may be required for unstable arrhythmias. Congenital QT syndrome is usually treated with beta blockers and, in high-risk patients, an implantable cardioverter-defibrillator.

74 i. This patient has a facial abscess with purulent drainage that is of dental origin. A tooth abscess, or root abscess, is an infection at the base of the tooth that may invade local bone and eventually surrounding soft tissue. The principal causes are untreated tooth decay, cracked teeth, or extensive periodontal disease. Main symptoms include pain, pressure or temperature sensitivity, and local swelling. Typically, the infection is due to nonpathologic bacteria already residing in the mouth, particularly gram-positive and anaerobic organisms.

ii. Penicillin remains the antibiotic of choice for the treatment of dental abscess, with clindamycin used in penicillin-allergic patients. Metronidazole can be added in complex cases. Incision and drainage of local abscesses is important, usually done intraorally. Occasionally, special imaging may be necessary to define the extent of the abscess.

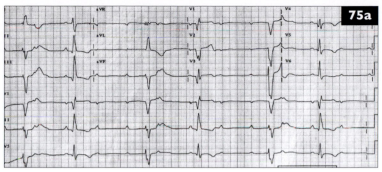

75 A 78-year-old male presented with new onset seizures. He reportedly had two 20-second generalized tonic–clonic seizures this morning, each with a postictal period of less than a minute. He had a past history of myocardial infarction and cerebrovascular accidents.

i. What does this ECG suggest (75a)?

ii. What treatment is recommended?

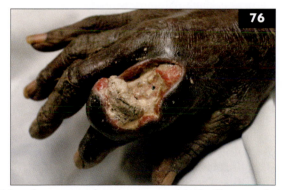

76 A 79-year-old male presented with a severe febrile illness and stated that he has had this problem with his hand for many months (76). The patient reported many previous episodes of intermittent severe joint pain in multiple joints, but he did not seek medical attention in the past because the problem always went away.

i. What do you think is going on?

ii. What evaluation and treatment does this patient need?

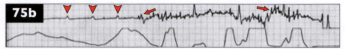

75 i. The history is atypical for simple seizures. Short episodes of epileptiform activity with minimal postictal period are often due to cerebral hypoperfusion. The ECG reveals complete heart block, with slow ventricular rate. (Periodic atrioventricular capture occurs in this case, with a different QRS complex.) The 'seizures' were actually myoclonic jerking due to cerebral ischemia. Complete heart block is a type of atrioventricular dissociation with atrial depolarizations not conducted and ventricular rhythm maintained by a secondary pacemaker. In infranodal third-degree block, ventricular rate is usually <40 bpm and regular, with wide QRS complex. Coronary ischemia and conduction system degeneration are common causes. Certain medications (e.g. beta blockers, calcium channel blockers), infections (e.g. Lyme disease), and cardiac surgeries are among other causes.

ii. Stabilization of complete heart block depends on perfusion status. If normal, simply monitor with transcutaneous pacing, if available, and consult cardiology. Hypoperfusion with third-degree heart block is best treated with transcutaneous pacing. Atropine or, less commonly, IV catecholamines (e.g. epinephrine) may be useful if pacing is not immediately available. This rhythm strip was recorded before transcutaneous pacing could be established (**75b**). Yes, this is ventricular asystole with residual P waves (arrowheads), along with myoclonic jerking, demonstrated by tremor artifact (arrows), due to brain ischemia!

76 i. This is a gouty tophus that has become huge and eroded through the skin. Diagnosis can be rapidly confirmed by microscopic analysis of lesion scrapings under polarized light, which revealed negatively birefringent needle-like crystals of monosodium urate. Gout is a metabolic disorder characterized by hyperuricemia due to overproduction or underexcretion of uric acid. Hyperuricemia leads to deposition of monosodium urate in joints and soft tissues, causing gouty arthritis and, over time, gouty tophi.

ii. Most important is to evaluate this patient for all potential sources of infection. A secondary local cellulitis is likely and appropriate antibiotic coverage may be indicated. Surgical debridement may also be necessary. Acute gouty attacks usually respond to NSAIDs, with colchicine an alternative if there are contraindications to that class of medications. Corticosteroids are also useful for acute exacerbations. Medications to prevent further episodes of gout include allopurinol, probenecid, and febuxostat, typically begun 1–2 weeks after symptom resolution (due to potential for worsening the attack).

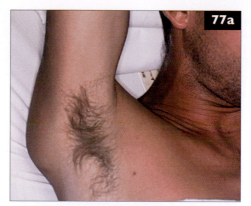

77 A 29-year old male fell about 3.7 m (12 feet) out of a tree and hurt his right shoulder, which he could not move from its present position (77a).
i. What do you think might be going on?
ii. How do you correct this problem?

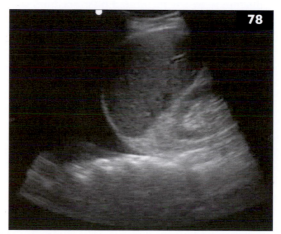

78 A 37-year-old male fell out of a two-story building and presented with severe chest pain and shortness of breath.
i. What does this right upper quadrant ultrasound image suggest (78)?
ii. How should he be managed?

77 i. This is luxatio erecta, an unusual (0.5%) inferior shoulder dislocation. It occurs when an axial load is placed on a fully abducted arm or when a hyperabducting force leverages the humeral head inferiorly out of the glenoid fossa. Associated bony fractures are common, particularly to the greater tuberosity of the humerus, as in this case (77b, arrow). Simple shoulder radiographs are usually adequate for evaluation. The

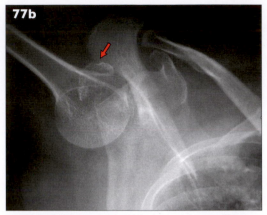

inferior joint capsule is always torn in luxatio erecta. Many have rotator cuff tears, injury to the axillary artery, as well as various nerve injuries.

ii. Search for associated injuries and perform a careful prereduction neurologic and vascular evaluation. Orthopedic consultation is appropriate, particularly with associated fractures, neurologic deficits, or evidence of vascular compromise. Traction on the hyperabducted arm, with the torso stabilized by an assistant, followed by adduction is the traditional reduction method. A two-step method has been described. Reduction is greatly facilitated by procedural sedation, but should usually only be attempted if orthopedic specialists are unavailable or with vascular compromise. Open reduction in the operating room is frequently required. Post-reduction radiographs and neurovascular examination are important. These patients are immobilized after reduction with a chest–arm bandage.

78 i. There is a normal hepatorenal space, but a significant quantity of fluid is visible in the right pleural space. In the setting of trauma, this is a traumatic hemothorax. This is an extended version of the ultrasound FAST examination, termed eFAST, which explores for hemothorax, pneumothorax, and intravascular filling status (by evaluating the inferior vena cava). The sensitivity and specificity of ultrasound for hemothorax are both very high.

ii. A thoracostomy tube should be inserted in the right pleural space to drain the accumulated blood. Drainage of over 1,500 ml acutely, 200–300 ml/hour for several hours, incomplete evacuation, or continued unstable vital signs thought secondary to pleural space bleeding are indications for emergency thoracotomy.

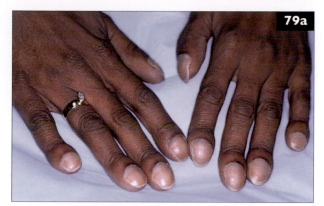

79 A 53-year-old female presented with a persistent cough over several weeks. She had this examination finding, which appeared over several months (79a).
i. What diseases are associated?
ii. How should she be evaluated?

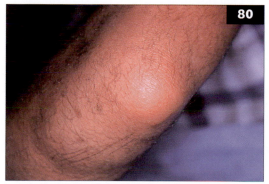

80 A 37-year-old male had painful swelling to his left elbow area after minor trauma (80). Radiographs of the area did not show bony injury.
i. What is this?
ii. How is this condition managed?

79 i. Clubbing of the fingers, also known as Hippocratic fingers among other names, is a deformity associated mostly with diseases of the heart and lungs. Any heart diseases featuring chronic hypoxia, along with infective endocarditis, are typical cardiac causes. Lung cancer causes over one-third of all cases of finger clubbing, with tuberculosis and suppurative lung diseases being other common

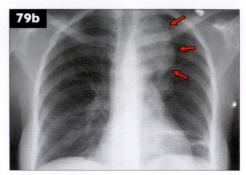

pulmonary etiologies. Many gastrointestinal causes exist and there are also familial and racial groups who appear to have increased frequency of clubbing. Cases are frequently idiopathic. Schamroth's test, in which distal phalanges of the corresponding fingers of opposite hands are placed fingernail to fingernail, is positive for clubbing if the normal diamond-shaped window is obliterated.
ii. Appropriate testing should be done based on expected etiologies. In this case chest radiography is appropriate, as a lung problem is most suggested. This revealed a left upper lobe mass (**79b**, arrows), which turned out to be squamous cell lung cancer.

80 i. Olecranon bursitis. Acute or repetitive trauma is the most common etiology, although crystalline joint disease (e.g. gout), chronic arthritis, or infection may be associated. This condition often results from repetitive minor elbow trauma. Focal swelling is the most common complaint, although olecranon bursitis is frequently painful, especially with infection. On examination, posterior elbow swelling is usually well demarcated and fluctuant. There may be local injury, erythema, and tenderness. Range of motion is generally normal, but often limited by pain with flexion. Make sure the elbow joint is not infected. There should be joint effusion and minimal range of motion with septic arthritis.
ii. Radiography should be done if significant associated trauma. Infection is suggested by previous local wound, cellulitis, redness, or fever. Bursal aspiration may be necessary, with a WBC count of 100×10^9/l ($100,000$/mm^3) or more in synovial fluid suggestive of infection. Gram staining with culture is useful to define causative organisms. Other laboratory tests are only needed to diagnose a related systemic illness (e.g. gout). If infection is suspected, appropriate antibiotics should be administered. For noninfectious olecranon bursitis, rest and NSAIDs are helpful. Local corticosteroid injection after aspiration may speed recovery and a compressive elbow dressing may reduce the rate of fluid reaccumulation.

81 A 45-year-old shopkeeper was shot once with a large caliber pistol during a robbery about 45 minutes prior to arrival. He presented awake and talking with BP of 92/68 mmHg (12.3/9.1 kPa), P 140 bpm, and RR 32/min. He had one wound in his right lateral antecubital fossa (**81a**) and, on careful inspection, no exit wound or other gunshot wound. He denied any other injuries. Para-

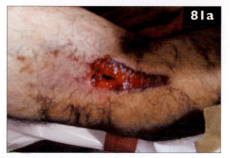

medics described a moderate amount of blood at the scene, but the wound was only oozing on arrival. He seemed to be deteriorating despite rapid infusion of 2 liters of normal saline.
i. What is going on here?
ii. What is the next step in management?

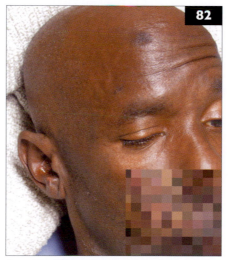

82 A 47-year-old male with AIDS had increased headaches recently with these findings (**82**).
i. What do you think is going on here?
ii. How should he be evaluated and managed?

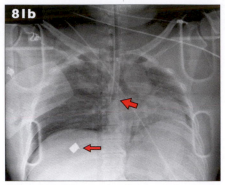

81 i. The original thought about this patient's clinical situation was that it was due to severe hemorrhage from the lateral antecubital fossa wound. However, with aggressive fluid resuscitation and absence of significant ongoing local bleeding, he should have improved rapidly. He did not. Understanding a bit of forensic medicine is important here. As it turns out, the shopkeeper was crouched down behind a counter with his arms up when the assailant shot down at him. The bullet traveled downward through his proximal arm and entered his right chest, where it caused considerable destruction.

ii. A chest radiograph (**81b**) revealed a bullet (thin arrow) in the right chest, and the full spectrum of injury was better understood. His right mainstem intubation (thick arrow) was recognized, and the endotracheal tube was pulled back. He failed to improve despite right thoracostomy tube placement, along with aggressive fluid and blood infusion, and underwent emergency thoracotomy.

82 i. The photograph suggests right peripheral facial nerve palsy, with right-sided loss of forehead wrinkling, subtle flattening of the nasolabial fold, and ptosis. Note associated rash in right ear canal and central pinna, defining Ramsay Hunt syndrome. Also known as geniculate neuralgia, Ramsay Hunt syndrome is an acute peripheral facial neuropathy associated with an erythematous, vesicular rash of the ear canal and auricle (herpes zoster oticus). It may be recurrent and is caused by varicella-zoster infection, sometimes latent in cranial nerves and dorsal root ganglia for many years. Occasionally, associated rash may be absent, with PCR of tear fluid showing virus. Fever, ear pain, unilateral hearing loss, tinnitus, and occasionally involvement of other cranial nerves, with related symptoms, may occur.

ii. CNS complications, including meningitis and encephalitis, may occur and are more common with HIV infections. CT scanning and lumbar puncture are indicated when associated CNS infection is suspected, with appropriate viral and other studies. Antiviral therapy (e.g. acyclovir) and corticosteroids are used, but not well studied in this disease. Pain management is important. Appropriate eye protection and lubrication is also necessary to prevent corneal injury, which may occur due to inadequate eye closure, particularly at night. Vestibular symptoms should be treated as necessary.

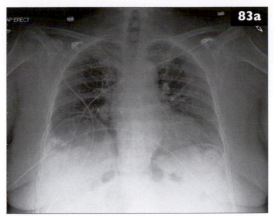

83 A 72-year-old female with a history of multiple medical problems presented with 5 days of fever along with a severe, nonproductive cough. She had some mild, diffuse abdominal tenderness on examination.
i. Are there any surprises on this chest radiograph (83a)?
ii. Does she need surgical intervention?

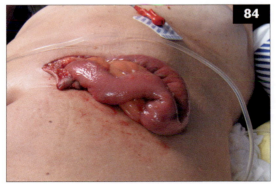

84 A 47-year-old bicyclist sustained this injury after she crashed and was impaled by a handlebar.
i. What are we seeing here (84)?
ii. How should this patient be managed?

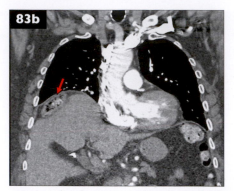

83 i. What might appear to be free air under the right hemidiaphragm, thus prompting a concern for surgical intervention, is actually something else. This is Chilaiditi's sign, an interposition of large bowel between the liver and diaphragm, often mistaken for pneumoperitoneum. It is more clearly defined by this CT image (**83b**, arrow). Chilaiditi's sign may be intermittent or permanent. It is found in asymptomatic patients and must be distinguished from Chilaiditi's syndrome, where there is associated symptomatology such as pain, respiratory distress, and bowel obstruction.

ii. No! This is Chilaiditi's sign, and the mild abdominal tenderness is much more likely musculoskeletal, probably due to muscular strain from prolonged cough. Chilaiditi's sign must be distinguished from pneumoperitoneum, which is usually due to gastrointestinal perforation unless some recent intervention has introduced intraperitoneal air.

84 i. A small intestine evisceration through a deep laceration in the anterior abdominal wall. Although the diagnosis is clear, this finding may distract from a careful and systematic trauma evaluation. Appropriate recognition of other injuries is occasionally missed when such a visible injury is present.

ii. Treatment of this injury includes covering the intestines with a moist sterile dressing, inserting a nasogastric tube for abdominal decompression, and immediate surgical consultation. Fluid losses may be significant with extensive intestinal prolapse. Broad-spectrum antibiotic coverage is indicated. Do not attempt to reduce the intestines back into the abdominal cavity before operating.

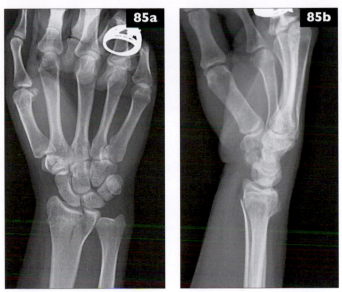

85 A 37-year-old female fell on her outstretched right hand and presented with severe wrist pain.
i. Discuss the issues with this injury (85a, b)?
ii. How should she be managed?

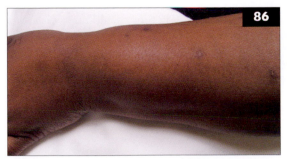

86 A 35-year-old female had been doing lots of lifting, carrying, and sweeping as well as other activities related to moving into a home. She presented with pain in the thumb side of her left wrist, which she thought was swollen.
i. What does this photograph suggest is a possible diagnosis (86)?
ii. What treatment is appropriate?

85 i. Distal radius fractures are the most frequent forearm bony injury, with the common mechanism being a fall on an outstretched hand (FOOSH). The classification of these fractures is based on direction of distal radius displacement, articular involvement, and associated injuries to ulna or carpal bones, as well as whether they are open or closed. A Colles' fracture is the most common distal radius break. It is a dorsally displaced fracture 2–3 cm from the radial articular surface, with associated ulnar styloid fracture in 50–60%. This patient's fracture is a bit more complex because there is intra-articular involvement. Acute associated complications include ulnar nerve injury, carpal tunnel syndrome, tendon injuries, pain, and hematoma. Plain radiographs are almost always adequate to evaluate distal radius fractures, with careful attention to alignment and articular involvement through multiple views.

ii. In younger patients, even 1 mm of joint surface incongruity leads to degenerative joint disease unless surgically repaired. This woman needs splinting, and orthopedic consultation within the next few days is necessary for definitive treatment.

86 i. There is dorsoradial swelling of the distal forearm from de Quervain's tenosynovitis (aka de Quervain's disease), an inflammation of the extensor pollicus brevis and abductor pollicus longus tendon areas. It is secondary to various repetitive activities involving the thumb and is frequent in mothers and day care workers who repetitively lift growing infants. Common etiologies include local trauma to the dorsoradial wrist as well as prolonged typing or use of personal communication devices. Tendons become inflamed in their sheaths. Local erythema, swelling, tenderness, and occasional crepitus with motion may be found along the distal dorsoradial wrist and thumb. The Finklestein test, done by flexing the thumb across the palm with deviation of the wrist ulnarly, causes substantial pain in de Quervain's tenosynovitis. Imaging is rarely indicated unless there is history of significant direct trauma.

ii. Splinting the thumb and wrist will improve symptoms, with rest and NSAIDs the mainstay of therapy. Local corticosteroid injections are frequently effective, but should be done by those experienced in the procedure. Surgical decompression of the first dorsal compartment will resolve symptoms for patients who fail more conservative therapies.

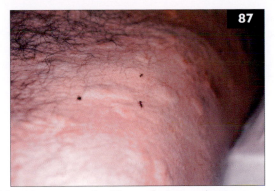

87 A 24-year-old male presented with confusion and agitation after being found unconscious in a ditch. BP was 64/40 mmHg (8.5/5.3 kPa), P 164 bpm, and RR 26/min. He had this pruritic rash (87).
i. What is the differential diagnosis, and how does this photograph help?
ii. How should he be treated?

88 A 39-year-old female fell while walking her dog and had pain in her left knee.
i. What does her radiograph suggest (88)?
ii. Are there criteria to help decide whether she even needed a radiograph?
iii. How should she be managed?

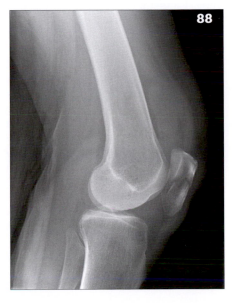

87 i. This patient is in shock. Differential diagnosis includes hypovolemic (e.g. volume loss, hemorrhage), cardiogenic (e.g. heart failure), obstructive (e.g. tension pneumothorax, pulmonary embolism, cardiac tamponade), or distributive (e.g. sepsis, anaphylaxis, neurogenic) types of shock. Urticaria here suggests anaphylactic shock, an acute multisystem hypersensitivity reaction to foreign protein, triggering release of immunologic mediators from mast cells and basophils, leading to vasodilation and mucosal edema. Yes, those are ants crawling on him! Urticaria, airway and peripheral angioedema, bronchospasm, abdominal cramps with vomiting and/or diarrhea, and cardiovascular collapse are common. Diagnosis requires recognition of clinical signs and symptoms, as no rapid laboratory tests are helpful. Eliciting history of exposure to medications (e.g. penicillin), stinging insects (e.g. fire ants), or foods (e.g. peanuts) that commonly trigger an allergic response may help. Often, the cause is unrecognized and nonimmunologic mechanisms (e.g. exercise-induced anaphylaxis) can precipitate this form of shock.
ii. Initial stabilization of severe anaphylactic shock includes supplemental oxygen with aggressive airway management, and rapid crystalloid infusion. Prompt use of epinephrine improves airway angioedema, stabilizes hemodynamics, and reduces mediator release. Appropriate dosing is not evidence based, but 10 ml of 1:10,000 in 250 ml of normal saline makes an epinephrine solution of about 4 mcg/ml, which can be titrated to symptom relief. Avoid subcutaneous or intramuscular dosing, because hypoperfusion may delay absorption. Antihistamines (e.g. diphenhydramine, 1 mg/kg), corticosteroids (e.g. methylprednisolone, 1–2 mg/kg), and liters of crystalloid may be needed.

88 i. A nondisplaced patellar fracture.
ii. The Ottawa knee rules are the most commonly used guidelines for knee injury patients. They suggest radiographic evaluation for knee trauma with any of the following: (1) age 55 years or older, (2) isolated patellar tenderness, (3) tenderness at the fibular head, (4) inability to flex to 90°, or (5) inability to bear weight both immediately or on medical evaluation (transferring weight twice onto each lower limb regardless of limping). Education is necessary concerning implementation of this rule, as patient expectations often drive radiographic evaluation. Most studies suggest use of the Ottawa knee rules will reduce radiography by about one-third without missing significant fractures.
iii. Fractures with intra-articular displacement >2 mm, with disrupted extensor mechanism, or those that are open require surgical treatment. Nondisplaced fractures, as here, may be treated by simple immobilization in a cylinder cast for 4–6 weeks.

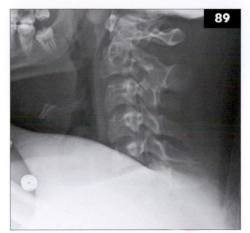

89 A 24-year-old female presented with severe neck pain after being an unrestrained front seat passenger who hit her forehead on the dashboard during a moderate-speed head-on collision. She was neurologically intact.
i. What does this lateral cervical spine view show (89)?
ii. Does this need surgical repair?

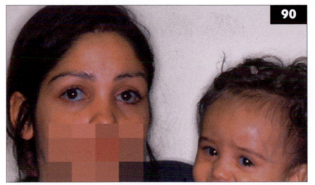

90 A 32-year-old female presented with these findings (90) and was concerned her child may have hurt something with a recent fall. The mother had multiple previous fractures.
i. What do you see in the photograph, and what is your differential diagnosis?
ii. Is there any treatment?

89 i. There is a bilateral pedicle fracture of the second cervical vertebrae (hangman's fracture). Although associated with judicial hangings, the primary mechanism of injury is forced hyperextension of the neck, often from the forehead striking the ground with a fall or the dashboard during a collision. On this lateral radiograph there is minimal anterior subluxation of the second vertebral body, while the posterior elements of C2 are clearly displaced posteriorly from the spinolaminar line. Note that this spinal view does not show a complete picture of all the cervical vertebrae, and further imaging is necessary to explore for associated injuries. Careful spine immobilization and thorough neurologic examination is necessary in all cases.

ii. Usually, this fracture may be managed with a halo vest device worn for about 3 months. Operative reduction with internal fixation is sometimes necessary, and orthopedic or neurosurgical consultation should always be engaged promptly.

90 i. In this situation we see blue sclera associated with osteogenesis imperfecta. Anything that causes scleral thinning may lead to a bluish discoloration, including aging, corticosteroid use, and iron deficiency. Many rare diseases of collagen (e.g. Marfan's syndrome) may have blue sclera. Osteogenesis imperfecta, or brittle bone disease, is a disorder of collagen associated with blue sclera, easily fractured bones, brittle teeth, scoliosis, short height, and hearing loss. Type I is the most common of at least eight types in one classification of osteogenesis imperfecta, and is the mildest. It is transmitted in an autosomal dominant manner. Severe cases of osteogenesis imperfecta may be recognized prenatally by ultrasound and can be diagnosed by biochemical or genetic testing.

ii. Fractures are evaluated in the usual manner, with surgical therapy frequently necessary. Biphosphonates have been found valuable in osteogenesis imperfecta by reducing bone pain, increasing bone density, and possibly reducing fracture incidence.

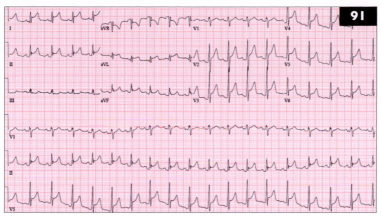

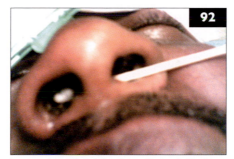

91 A 32-year-old male presented with severe chest pain of 4-hours duration. He had no previous medical history.
i. What does this ECG reveal (**91**)?
ii. What treatment is recommended?

92 A 34-year-old male presented with this clinical finding (**92**). He was very agitated, with a BP of 220/124 mmHg (29.3/16.5 kPa), P 148 bpm, RR 32/min, and T 38.6°C. What is the likely etiology?

91 i. Diffuse concave ST segment elevations, with PR segment depression in multiple leaves, consistent with acute pericarditis. The most common recognized cause is infection, usually viral, but occasionally by bacteria (including tuberculosis), parasites, and fungi. Malignancy, autoimmune illnesses (e.g. systemic lupus erythematosus), uremia, drug-related, postmyocardial infarction, and idiopathic causes are other considerations. Acute pericarditis may present with chest pain, typically pleuritic and improved by leaning forward. Fever and shortness of breath are common. You may hear a pericardial friction rub, a scratchy sound with 1–3 components that is frequently transient. Pericardial tamponade may be present, often with jugular venous distension, tachycardia, and/or hypotension. ECG changes in pericarditis have four stages: (1) most suggestive and involves diffuse, concave ST segment elevations and PR segment depressions; (2) ST segments return to baseline with T wave flattening; (3) exhibits diffuse T wave inversion, which gradually resolves in the fourth stage. Ultrasound or echocardiography should exclude pericardial effusion and/or tamponade, particularly with tachycardia and/or hypotension. Cardiac enzymes are frequently elevated due to associated myocarditis. Occasionally, myopericarditis mimics acute myocardial infarction.
ii. Treatment starts with management of the underlying disease, when recognized. NSAIDs are the initial therapy of choice, resolving symptoms within days in 85–90%. Colchicine reduces incidence of recurrent pericarditis. Corticosteroids are reserved for treatment failure from NSAIDs. Drainage procedures are indicated for pericardial effusion with tamponade.

92 This is a nasal septal perforation, a hole or fissure through the cartilaginous tissue. This can be intentional with nasal piercings, but also seen with traumatic injury, chronic use of vasoconstrictive or steroid nasal sprays, collagen vascular diseases (e.g. Wegener's granulomatosis), infectious diseases (e.g. syphilis), malignancy, certain other medications (e.g. bevacizumab), and chronic cocaine use. In this patient in a severe hyperadrenergic state, cocaine intoxication seems very likely. Surgical techniques exist for repair of septal perforation, if desired.

93 A 57-year-old female presented with 2 days of diffuse, crampy abdominal pain and severe diarrhea. BP was 96/64 mmHg (12.8/8.5 kPa) and P 136 bpm. She was recently treated for 'bronchitis with some antibiotic'.
i. What is likely to be the problem?
ii. How should she be treated?

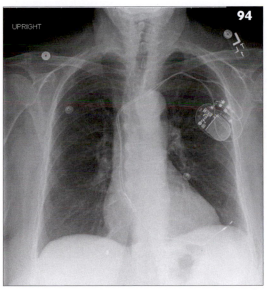

94 A 80-year-old female had a cardiac pacemaker placed 1 week ago and reported 2 days of pleuritic left upper abdominal and lower chest pain along with increased burping.
i. What does this chest radiograph show (**94**)?
ii. Does anything need to be done?

93 i. Antibiotic-associated diarrhea due to indiscriminate use of antibiotics. This is usually mild, self-limiting, due to intestinal flora changes, and resolves with supportive care and discontinuation of antibiotics. However, a small percentage of patients with broad-spectrum antibiotic therapy, particularly extended-spectrum penicillins, cephalosporins, or clindamycin, develop diarrhea due to overgrowth of *Clostridium difficile*. Risk factors include advanced age, immunocompromised state, recent abdominal surgery, prolonged antibiotic use, extended hospital stay, recent use of proton pump inhibitors, and other comorbidities. Patients may present with symptoms that vary from mild diarrhea to fulminant colitis. Colonoscopy in severe cases reveals extensive areas of colonic mucosal erythema and ulcers with overlying sheets of exudates, leading to the term pseudomembranous colitis. Diagnosis is confirmed by identification of *C. difficile* toxin in stool using PCR, ELISA, cultures, or much less specific latex agglutination tests.

ii. Treatment begins with fluid and electrolyte replacement along with discontinuation of antibiotics. Give oral metronidazole when diagnosis of *C. difficile* colitis is confirmed, or empirically in ill patients when likely. Vancomycin is preferred in young children, pregnancy, and/or with metronidazole intolerance or failure. It is also appropriate in critically ill patients or if metronidazole resistance is likely. In severe cases, relapse occurs in 15–20%.

94 i. Pacemaker lead perforation of the right ventricular wall. This is a rare complication of lead placement and may present with pericardial tamponade, device failure, syncope, chest or abdominal pain, or be completely asymptomatic. Atrial lead perforations are more common than ventricular ones, and both are more common with active fixation leads. ECG may show pacing failure. Imaging of lead perforation includes chest radiography, CT, or echocardiography. The pleuritic pain and increased burping were likely secondary to abnormal electrical stimulations from the displaced pacemaker lead.

ii. Echocardiography should be done to exclude pericardial effusion and/or tamponade. Simple lead repositioning or replacement under fluoroscopic guidance, with surgical back-up, is usually successful.

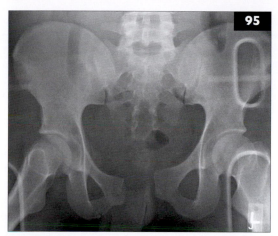

95 A 67-year-old male presented with mainly lower abdominal and pelvic pain following a motor vehicle collision. BP was 90/64 (12.0/8.5 kPa) with P 140 bpm.
i. What does this radiograph suggest (95)?
ii. Assuming no other injuries are found, what is the management of this problem?

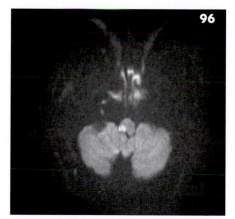

96 A 47-year-old male presented with sudden onset of nausea and vomiting along with ataxia and double vision. He had no focal neurologic deficits on examination.
i. What does this diffusion-weighted MR image suggest (96)?
ii. What treatment is indicated?

95 i. The radiograph reveals a widened pubic symphysis, right inferior ramus fracture, and subtle disruption of the right sacroiliac joint. Multiple classification systems of pelvic fractures exist. The complication rate is significant, mainly related to associated organ injuries and bleeding. On examination, tenderness or instability on palpation is suggestive of fracture, but repetitive examinations should be avoided as movement may increase bleeding. Hematuria, hematochezia, or vaginal bleeding in females may be associated. Anteroposterior radiographs uncover most pelvic fractures, while CT shows more detail and helps recognize significant associated injuries.

ii. Most pelvic fractures represent significant trauma and evaluation for associated injuries is important. Provide aggressive volume resuscitation, appropriate trauma blood studies, and early blood transfusion when indicated. Bladder catheterization may be necessary. However, if hematuria or other evidence of lower urinary tract injury exists, catheterization should be preceded by an urethrogram (in males) followed by a cystogram. Pelvic fractures are associated with more injury than suggested by plain radiography, as recoil from displacement prevents recognition of how much tissue was stretched and torn. Application of an external compression device to an unstable pelvis will provide mechanical stabilization and help control hemorrhage. Binding with a sheet or one of several commercial products is effective. Interventional radiology for vessel embolization may be necessary to further control bleeding. Prompt orthopedic consultation is important to provide definitive repair.

96 i. Infarction in the right lateral medulla, which causes posterior inferior cerebellar artery syndrome (PICA), also called lateral medullary or Wallenberg's syndrome. It is one of the most commonly recognized neurologic conditions due to brainstem infarct. Frequent symptoms include dysphonia, dysphagia, diplopia, and ataxia. Ipsilateral facial pain and/or numbness, with loss of pain and temperature sensation on the opposite side of the body, are the complaints usually bringing this specific diagnosis to mind, but are present infrequently. PICA syndrome is most commonly caused by vertebral artery or a branch occlusion, sometimes due to traumatic dissection. MRI with special imaging techniques is the best way to confirm the diagnosis, and MRA may help define arterial involvement.

ii. Treatment is supportive, with attention to speech and swallowing retraining. Antiepileptic medications may help with chronic pain.

97 A 21-year-old male was un-helmeted when he crashed his moped into a vehicle and hit his right face on the ground. His right cheek was sore and it hurt to open his mouth.
i. What does this photograph suggest (97a)?
ii. What is the appropriate management?

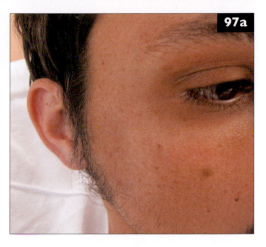

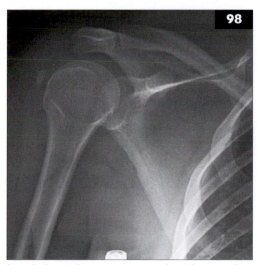

98 A 44-year-old female housekeeper presented with 2 weeks of increasing right shoulder pain, which was worse with movement. There was no history of trauma.
i. What does this radiograph suggest (98)?
ii. How should the problem be treated?

97 i. The photograph shows a subtle depression over the right zygomatic arch, suggesting a depressed fracture there. The zygomatic arch overlies the temporalis muscle and the coronoid process of the mandible. With traumatic depression, jaw opening becomes limited and painful. The zygomatic arch also is an important aesthetic component of the face. The facial depression, barely seen here, is often not visible due to hematoma and edema secondary to the fracture, and this may delay recognition.

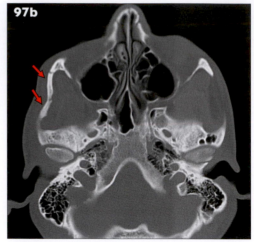

ii. CT may better define zygomatic arch fractures and associated injuries (**97b**). This fracture (arrows) will require surgical elevation and mechanical stabilization, which can be done in a delayed fashion.

98 i. Calcific tendinitis of the shoulder, characterized by deposits of hydroxyapatite crystals in any tendon of the rotator cuff. The supraspinatus tendon is affected most often. Shoulder calcific tendonitis is rarely associated with rotator cuff tears and is frequently asymptomatic. When symptomatic, it usually causes mild, intermittent shoulder pain exacerbated by repetitive activities. Only rarely does calcific tendonitis block shoulder movement. Plain radiographs are usually adequate for diagnosis.

ii. Nonoperative management is successful in most patients. Spontaneous resorption is common. Rest and physical therapy are often all that is necessary for improvement. NSAIDs are commonly prescribed. Needle aspiration and lavage of calcific material may be effective in skilled hands. Corticosteroid and local anesthetic injections, as well as extracorporeal shock wave therapy, have some utility. Surgical therapy, by open or arthroscopic techniques, is frequently successful in severe cases.

99 A 52-year-old male with end-stage renal disease presented after hemodialysis with severe muscle cramps that lasted a few minutes at a time and moved from the back to the extremities. He was in severe pain.
i. What is the problem, and what is the likely cause?
ii. How should this be treated?

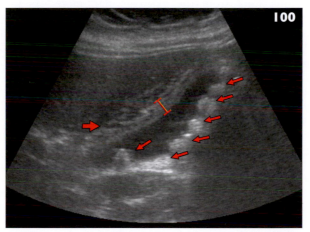

100 A 47-year-old female presented with recurrent, postprandial, right upper quadrant and back pain with nausea and vomiting. She had been hurting in her right upper abdomen for several hours today and had recent fever with chills. On examination, her T was 39.2°C. She appeared to have subtle scleral icterus and was tender in her right upper quadrant.
i. What does this ultrasound image suggest (100)?
ii. What should be considered here?
iii. What therapy is indicated?

99 i. Muscle cramps are a frequent complication of hemodialysis treatment, occurring in a third or more of these patients. Although the exact etiology of muscle cramps in dialysis patients is unknown, changes in plasma osmolality and/or extracellular fluid volume seem to correlate. Electrolyte imbalances may be a component of the problem. These muscle cramps can be severe and tend to occur near the end of or shortly after hemodialysis, often contributing to undertreatment.
ii. Management of hemodialysis-related muscle cramps is simple. Although volume replacement with normal saline IV seems appropriate, this may obviate the fluid removal dialysis accomplished. Other techniques to increase intravascular volume are more sensible. Small infusions of hyperosmotic agents, particularly concentrated dextrose solutions (e.g. dextrose 50% in water), increase intravascular volume rapidly by pulling fluid from the extravascular space. As the dextrose is metabolized, the intravascular volume tends to gradually normalize, while the early increased muscle perfusion resolves the muscle cramps. IV mannitol and hypertonic saline have also been used for hemodialysis-related muscle spasms. Do not forget appropriate pain medication!

100 i. The ultrasound shows multiple gallstones (thin arrows), a thickened gallbladder wall (lines), and a small amount of pericholecystic fluid (thick arrow), very suggestive of acute cholecystitis.
ii. Charcot's triad: jaundice, right upper quadrant pain, and fever. Although quite suggestive of acute cholangitis, all three components are present in less than a quarter of patients with this problem, with fever in 90%, abdominal pain in 70%, and jaundice in 60%. If hypotension and altered mental status also exist, this constitutes Reynolds' pentad, which makes acute cholangitis extremely likely. Choledocholithiasis is the most common cause of acute cholangitis, although it may also occur with local tumors or after endoscopic retrograde cholangiopancreatography (ERCP). Acute cholangitis is a bacterial infection superimposed on biliary tract obstruction. Common causative organisms are *Escherichia coli*, *Klebsiella*, *Enterococcus*, and *Pseudomonas* species.
iii. Acute cholangitis has high mortality if not appropriately managed. Early volume resuscitation is important along with broad-spectrum antibiotics to cover likely causative organisms. Except in mild cases without evidence of sepsis, emergency decompression of the biliary tree is important. This may be accomplished by percutaneous, endoscopic, or surgical drainage, with ERCP still the mainstay of therapy in many areas. Prompt surgical and/or gastroenterology consultation is important.

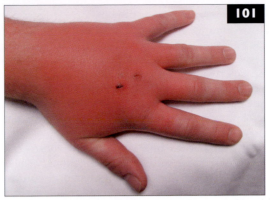

101 A 29-year-old male animal groomer was bitten by one of his feline clients about 20 hours prior to presentation. He arrived with these painful skin changes (101), but was able to move all of his fingers and his wrist normally.
i. What does this photograph suggest (101)?
ii. How should he be managed?

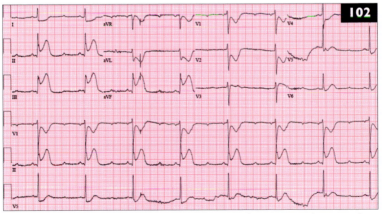

102 A 49-year-old male presented with severe chest pain along with nausea, diaphoresis, and hypotension. He had no known previous medical problems.
i. What does the ECG show (102)?
ii. How should this patient be managed?

101 i. There are small puncture wounds on the dorsal hand consistent with cat bites, along with surrounding erythema due to cellulitis. Certain organisms are likely culprits in cat bites and scratches, particularly *Pasteurella* species. The hand has many structures with decreased vascularity that are easily inoculated by razor-sharp cat teeth, particularly tendon, joint, and bone. A careful examination should be done to exclude these infectious complications.

ii. Confirm that the cat had appropriate rabies vaccinations, although this bite certainly would be classified as a provoked attack. Irrigation and debridement of devitalized tissue may be useful in fresh wounds, but not here. The goal of antibiotic therapy (and prophylaxis if an early bite) is to cover *Streptococcus*, *Staphylococcus*, *Pasteurella*, and anaerobic species. Antibiotic therapy should be broad spectrum, with amoxicillin–clavulanate a good first choice. Other oral regimens might include clindamycin or cephalexin plus either a fluoroquinolone or trimethoprim–sulfamethoxazole. Infections complicated by tenosynovitis, joint or bone infection, and any immunocompromised state likely will require aggressive IV antibiotic therapy. Make sure to address tetanus immunization status and provide pain control. Careful follow-up of cat bite infections is important, as complications are common.

102 i. 3:1 atrioventricular block and a narrow-complex ventricular escape rate at about 48 bpm. The inferior leads (II, III, and aVF) show 3–5 mm of ST elevation, with 2–3 mm of ST depression in the lateral (I, aVL, V_5, and V_6) and septal (V_1 and V_2) leads. This is evidence of acute inferior wall myocardial infarction with reciprocal changes, although concomitant septal ischemia is also likely. The atrioventricular block is probably due to increased vagal tone or atrioventricular nodal ischemia. Intranodal block usually has a narrow QRS complex and a ventricular rate of 40–60 bpm.

ii. Appropriate attention to ABC is important. Supplemental oxygen plus bolus IV fluids have priority. About 40% of inferior wall myocardial infarctions involve the right ventricle, and rapidly infused crystalloid may be necessary to restore perfusion. If fluid boluses do not quickly improve the hemodynamic status, rate improvement with atropine and/or transcutaneous pacing may help. Vasopressor therapy (e.g. norepinephrine) may be necessary if the previous measures do not restore adequate perfusion. This patient is a candidate for immediate reperfusion therapy, with percutaneous coronary intervention preferred over thrombolytics. Standard therapies for acute coronary syndrome, including aspirin and heparin (also glycoprotein 2b3a inhibitors if percutaneous intervention is planned), are among the clearly indicated interventions.

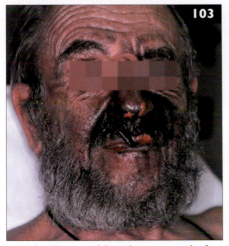

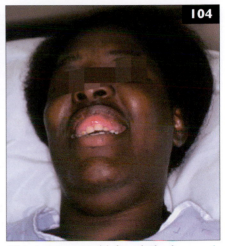

103 A 64-year-old male presented after an accident at home (103).
i. What do you think happened to him?
ii. What concerns should we have?

104 A 24-year-old female had a particular neurologic disorder for which she used a certain medication, but she could not remember its name. Does this photograph suggest the medication (104)?

105 A 29-year-old female presented with a new-onset, generalized, tonic–clonic seizure that began 8 minutes prior to arrival. She had a history of Sheehan's syndrome (postpartum pituitary apoplexy) and recently was placed on amoxicillin for a new diagnosis of pneumonia. She was on levothyroxine, prednisone, and low-dose estrogen, which she had been taking without any recent change in dosing.
i. What is important to consider here?
ii. How should she be treated?

103 i. A hint to the mechanism is recognition of a blackened piece of oxygen tubing hanging from his right philtrum area and nose. Yes, he was smoking while receiving supplemental oxygen and sustained thermal burns to his face.

ii. Besides the obvious concern that this patient might not understand the basics of combustion, these thermal burns must be taken seriously. Gentle cleaning with soap and water may reveal them to be deeper than is obvious and, depending on what exactly happened, the airway may also be injured more extensively. Supplemental oxygen and airway evaluation, possibly by laryngoscopic or fiberoptic visualization, is necessary. Early endotracheal intubation may be required if there is evidence of thermal injury in the hypopharynx and beyond, as mucosal thickening and edema may greatly complicate delayed airway management.

104 This patient has gum hypertrophy, which is a frequent complication of phenytoin, a common antiepileptic medication. Other medications associated with gum hypertrophy include cyclosporine and nifedipine. It is also seen in lead and arsenic poisoning as well as some leukemias, pregnancy, scurvy, and poor oral hygiene.

105 i. Infection increases metabolic stress, which for those on chronic low-dose corticosteroid therapy may lead to secondary adrenal insufficiency. Normally, stress triggers increased adrenal corticosteroid release up to tenfold, allowing management of higher metabolic demands. With long-term corticosteroid use, the hypothalamic–pituitary axis is suppressed and adrenal glands atrophy. Only increased supplemental corticosteroids allow avoidance of acute adrenal insufficiency, which presents with nausea, vomiting, abdominal pain, muscle weakness and fatigue, hypotension, hypothermia, and variable alterations in mental status, including seizures. Laboratory tests may show hyperkalemia, hyponatremia, hypoglycemia, and low serum cortisol. This patient's serum glucose was 0.44 mmol/l (8 mg/dl). Early glucose measurement is appropriate in most presentations involving altered mental status of unknown etiology.

ii. Immediate dextrose infusion is necessary. Supplemental corticosteroids resolve the adrenal crisis, with optimal dosing not studied. Up to 250 mg hydrocortisone/day or equivalent is typically used. Address critical levels of hyponatremia and/or hyperkalemia, although corticosteroids alone correct these electrolyte abnormalities over time. With hypoperfusion, mineralocorticoid replacement may be necessary (e.g. fludrocortisone) in addition to aggressive crystalloid infusion. Chronic corticosteroid users with significant infections or other stressors should usually increase their replacement therapy by 3–4 times over normal daily maintenance doses until the problem resolves.

106 A 54-year-old male presented with pleuritic chest pain, nonproductive cough, and fever that had not responded to 5 days of azithromycin therapy. He smoked one pack of cigarettes daily and had recent skin grafting to his leg for burns. BP was 96/60 mmHg (12.8/8.0 kPa), P 102 bpm, RR 18/min, T 38.6°C, and P$_{ox}$ 97%.

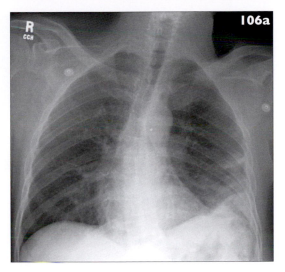

i. Any thoughts about this chest radiograph and this patient (106a)?
ii. What other therapy would you suggest?

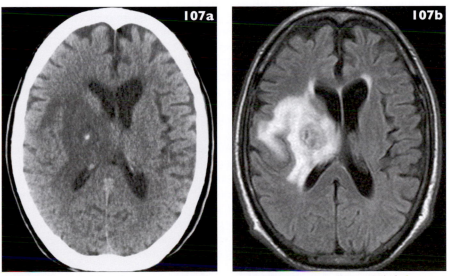

107 A 67-year-old male presented with an unsteady gait as well as subtle left upper and lower extremity weakness. He had a distant history of lung malignancy.
i. What do his head CT scan (107a) and MR image suggest (107b)?
ii. How could this be managed?

106 i. Maybe this is still pneumonia, but the chest radiograph seems to show only atelectasis with an elevated left hemidiaphragm. We probably need to expand our differential diagnosis and with the recent burns and surgery, pulmonary embolism must rise to the top of the list. Hypotension and fever, though less common, both occur with blood clots to the lung. A chest CT angiogram (**106b**) certainly is indicated, and it shows multiple pulmonary emboli (arrows) with left lung atelectasis.

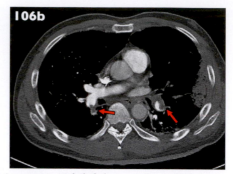

106b

ii. Heparin therapy is indicated, with IV unfractionated heparin or subcutaneous enoxaparin appropriate. Thrombolytics have no proven mortality or morbidity advantage and may be even less effective in these pulmonary clots, which have likely been in the pulmonary vasculature several days, are partly organized by fibroblasts, and thus less easily lysed.

107 i. There is a large right medial temporoparietal hypodense area, lateral ventricle effacement, and slight midline shift. The punctate central hyperdensity may represent hemorrhage. MRI often reveals complementary information. The most common intracranial tumor in adults is metastasis from systemic cancer (lung, breast, melanoma, renal, and colon in order of decreasing frequency). Lung cancer and melanoma often have multiple metastases. About 85% of metastases are to the cerebrum, with 15% to the cerebellum or brainstem. Symptoms relate to tumor location, with headache, often most severe on awakening, and seizure the two most common complaints. New onset seizure in older patients is frequently due to a brain tumor. About one-third with brain metastases exhibit motor and/or cognitive deficits. Tumor edema frequently contributes to neurologic deficit, often causing morning exacerbations. Acute tumor hemorrhage may create abrupt presentations in previously asymptomatic patients.

ii. Early diagnosis and treatment of brain metastases has increased survival. Head elevation to 30–45°, along with IV dexamethasone, reduces brain edema. Treat seizures with typical antiepileptic medications (e.g. phenytoin), with prophylaxis unnecessary if no prior seizure. Radiation therapy is the main treatment of brain metastases. Neurosurgery is reserved for solitary lesions larger than 3 cm in non-essential brain areas with a functional patient whose systemic cancer is controlled. Chemotherapy, usually in conjunction with radiation therapy and surgery, may prolong survival in some tumor types (e.g. small cell lung, lymphoma, and breast).

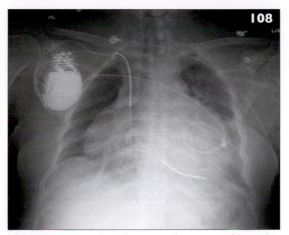

108 A 62-year-old male presented with severe shortness of breath and lightheaded-ness. He had a pacemaker placed 9 days ago. BP was 68/40 mmHg (9.1/5.3 kPa), P 112 bpm, and RR 32/min. Medications included coumadin and lisinopril.
i. What does this chest radiograph suggest (**108**)?
ii. What tests will be immediately important?

109 An 80 kg, 27-year-old male with severe asthma required intubation and paralysis with mechanical ventilation after multiple nebulized treatments with inhaled beta agonists and anticholinergics, high-dose parenteral corticosteroids, and IV magnesium failed to resolve his severe respiratory distress. His respirator settings were intermittent mandatory ventilation with RR 16/min, tidal volume of 1,200 cm^3 (15 cm^3/kg) per breath, and positive end expiratory pressure (PEEP) of 5 mmHg (0.7 kPa). He quickly became hypotensive and very tachycardic.
i. What is the cause of his hemodynamic deterioration?
ii. What should be done?

108 i. The chest radiograph is a bit complex. It shows a very large, globular heart (although the radiograph is slightly rotated). There is a pacemaker-defibrillator with three leads, including a right atrial and right ventricular IV lead as well as a left ventricular epicardial lead. There is no strong evidence for pulmonary edema.

ii. Immediate cardiac ultrasound or echocardiogram is necessary to assess for pericardial tamponade, which was present here. It was thought to be due to an intracardiac lead that perforated the right ventricle and led to progressive bleeding. Checking the prothrombin time is also important, with correction indicated if significantly anticoagulated. The patient was taken to surgery for an immediate pericardial window.

109 i. Several potential causes of hypoperfusion exist. Medications used in rapid sequence intubation (here ketamine and succinylcholine) cause a sympatholysis. Asthma patients are often dehydrated due to lack of oral intake, with increased insensible losses from sweating and respiratory efforts. However, the most important consideration here is termed intrinsic PEEP, also known as auto-PEEP or breath stacking. Remember, the main breathing problem in many respiratory illnesses is difficulty with lung emptying. Auto-PEEP is defined as an increase in end-expiratory intrapulmonary pressure resulting from dynamic airflow resistance during mechanical ventilation, directly related to lung hyperinflation. Risk factors may be intrinsic (thickened secretions, airway narrowing) or extrinsic (small endotracheal tube, high minute ventilation). In this case both tidal volume and RR are too high. Air trapping raises intrathoracic pressure and reduces venous return to the heart, contributing to hypotension and tachycardia. Although barotrauma (e.g. tension pneumothorax), myocardial ischemia, and even succinylcholine-induced hyperkalemia are other possible causes of hypotension, the possibility of auto-PEEP must be dealt with first.

ii. This patient's hypoperfusion needs rapid definitive action. Immediately disconnect the ventilator, with gentle pressure applied to the central chest to help empty the lung of excess air over 20–30 seconds. If auto-PEEP is the etiology of hypoperfusion, there should be rapid hemodynamic improvement. Re-establish ventilation using tidal volume of 6–8 ml/kg, RR of 6–8/min, and a high inspiratory flow rate. This is termed permissive hypercapnea or controlled hypoventilation, which has been shown to reduce mortality in intubated patients with asthma and COPD. If hemodynamic improvement does not occur, the other etiologies discussed above must be considered.

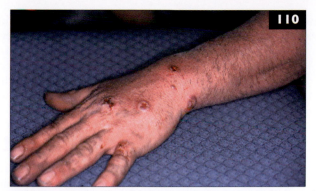

110 A 35-year-old homeless male presented with these painful ulcers (**110**), which had spread over several days.
i. What is this rash, and what causes it?
ii. What are the basics of therapy for this condition?

111 A 58-year-old male was angry and violent this morning for unclear reasons, which resolved on its own. He later became confused again and was sent to the hospital. He had hypertension and diabetes mellitus treated with furosemide, metoprolol, lisinopril, glyburide, and pioglitazone. Four days ago, he was placed on levofloxacin for a urinary tract infection. He was fully alert on presentation and neurologically intact. BP was 140/84 mmHg (18.7/11.2 kPa), P 64 bpm, RR 18/min, T 37.8°C, and blood glucose 3.1 mmol/l (56 mg/dl).
i. What do you think is going on in this case?
ii. What should be done?

110 i. Ecthyma, an ulcerative pyoderma of the skin that is similar to impetigo, but penetrates into the dermis. It is caused primarily by group A beta-hemolytic streptococci. It can be seen in areas of previous skin injury (e.g. wounds, insect bites), particularly in hot, humid, and crowded environments, often in patients with poor hygiene. It is more common in diabetes mellitus, HIV, and other immuno-compromised conditions. Ecthyma begins as a pustule or vesicle over inflamed skin and progresses to a deep dermal ulcer with crusting and raised, indurated margins. Ulcers may grow to several centimeters in diameter and are painful. Lymph-adenopathy is common. Cellulitis, lymphangitis, and, rarely, bacteremia with systemic illness may occur. Ecthyma heals with local scarring.

ii. Treatment begins with local wound care. Soap cleansing and efforts to remove wound crusting using warm compresses are important. Antibacterial ointments may be adequate for localized ecthyma. Penicillin therapy is effective for more extensive ecthyma, although antistaphylococcal agents (e.g. cephalexin, trimethoprim–sulfomethoxazole) are often added to cover secondary infections with *Staphylococcus aureus*.

111 i. The likely problem here is drug-induced hypoglycemia as the cause of intermittent altered mental status. Sulfonylureas (particularly chlorpropamide and glyburide) are the most frequent triggers for medication-induced hypoglycemia not due to insulin. Many situations increase the risk of sulfonylurea-induced hypoglycemia including accidental overdose, increased age, decreased caloric intake, increased exercise, and various drug interactions. Here, the initiation of levofloxacin, or any quinolone, reduces the metabolism of glyburide and potentiates its effect. Several antibiotic classes and many other medications potentiate sulfonylureas, and one must be careful when adding anything to a diabetic regimen. Beta blockade (e.g. metoprolol) also reduces the sympathomimetic response to hypoglycemia.

ii. At the least, a prolonged period of observation is necessary to recognize and manage recurrent hypoglycemia. Levofloxacin should be stopped. A urinalysis should be done and an alternative, thoughtfully selected antibiotic prescribed if urinary tract infection still exists. (**Note:** It is also possible intermittent bacteremia could have caused this altered mental status.) Remember to check for medication interactions. A meal should be provided. If severe sulfonylurea-induced hypo-glycemia occurs and cannot be managed with IV dextrose, octreotide is useful to reverse hypoglycemia.

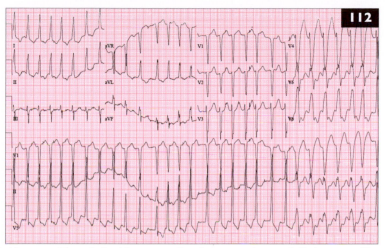

112 A 42-year-old male had longstanding hypertension and diabetes mellitus with two previous myocardial infarctions. He presented with severe chest tightness, palpitations, and shortness of breath. BP was 96/60 mmHg (12.8/8.0 kPa) with P 176 bpm.
i. What is going on here (112)?
ii. How should he be treated?

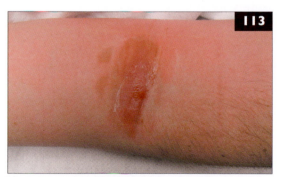

113 A 19-year-old male presented with 1 day of swelling and redness in his right antecubital fossa. He reluctantly admitted to IV heroin use. BP was 144/80 mmHg (19.1/10.7 kPa) with P 84 bpm, RR 18/min, and T 38.4°C.
i. What does this photograph suggest (113), and is there anything to worry about here?
ii. How should he be evaluated and managed?

112 i. Atrial fibrillation with a rapid ventricular response. It is interesting that the six beats before the last beat are wide-complex with a left bundle branch block pattern. This is probably simply a short run of rate-related bundle branch block, as it too is irregular. It is easy at high rates not to recognize the irregularity of atrial fibrillation.

ii. This patient must be assumed to have ongoing acute coronary syndrome. Rate reduction will decrease myocardial oxygen consumption, increase diastolic coronary perfusion time, and may improve BP as well as systemic perfusion. However, this patient with rapid atrial fibrillation and ongoing chest discomfort with hypotension needs prompt, safe therapy. Most medications used to treat atrial fibrillation will further reduce BP and may lead to cardiac arrest. Immediate electrical cardioversion is the appropriate treatment here. If neither chest pain nor significant hypotension were present, IV beta blockers (particularly esmolol with its short half-life) or calcium channel blockers (e.g. diltiazem) are reasonable choices. Class Ic (e.g. propafenone) and Class III (e.g. amiodarone) antiarrhythmics are often successful at converting atrial fibrillation to sinus rhythm; however, in this clinical situation, electricity is the 'drug of choice'.

113 i. The photograph suggests cellulitis in the antecubital fossa and beyond. Gathering the history of injectable drug use was important. Repeated venipunctures, needle sharing, and injection of insoluble materials are some of the issues that predispose IV drug users to complicated infections. Cellulitis may coexist with abscesses, pseudoaneurysms, and thrombosed veins. Infections are frequently polymicrobial, although *Staphylococcus aureus* and streptococcal species are the main culprits.

ii. Special imaging by ultrasound, CT, or MRI is often appropriate to exclude associated pathology. Careful inspection and often needle aspiration or incision may be necessary to define clearly the extent of infection and to drain abscesses. This patient had a substantial underlying abscess and tissue necrosis. As is often the case with infections in IV drug abusers, hospitalization with broad-spectrum antibiotics, along with repeated debridement, was necessary.

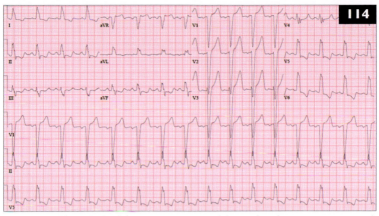

114 A 63-year-old male had hypertension and hyperlipidemia. He presented with severe chest pain and shortness of breath. BP was 140/94 mmHg (18.7/12.5 kPa) with P 84 bpm.
i. What does this ECG suggest (**114**)? (There is no previous ECG for comparison.)
ii. What intervention is indicated?

115 A 78-year-old male presented with severe abdominal pain and distension, but no vomiting or diarrhea. Abdominal radiography was performed (**115**).
i. What is the diagnosis?
ii. What is the initial management?

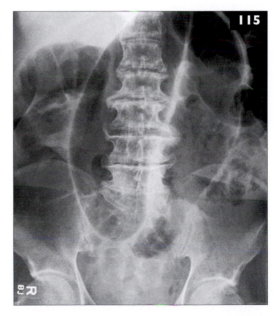

114 i. The ECG shows NSR with ventricular rate about 92 bpm and left bundle branch block (LBBB). We must assume this LBBB is new, which is a criterion for acute STEMI management. Sgarbossa described three criteria to assist in detection of myocardial infarction in patients with LBBB: (1) ST segment elevation greater than or equal to 1 mm concordant with the QRS complex in any lead, (2) ST segment elevation greater than or equal to 5 mm discordant with the QRS complex in any lead, and (3) ST segment depression in leads V_1 to V_3. In particular, ST segment elevation concordant with the QRS complex has a high likelihood ratio for identification of acute myocardial infarction in LBBB, with criterion 2 above also fairly useful.

ii. The history suggests acute coronary syndrome, and with presumed new LBBB, immediate percutaneous coronary intervention is indicated. Do not forget standard therapies for acute coronary syndrome.

115 i. Sigmoid volvulus, an abnormal colonic twisting causing proximal obstruction. It can cause strangulation and necrosis of involved segments. Sigmoid volvulus is a common cause of intestinal obstruction, particularly in the elderly. It is frequent and occurs at a younger age in South America, Africa, and parts of Asia where consumption of high-fiber diet leads to redundant sigmoid colon. Predisposing factors include chronic constipation, megacolon, and an excessively mobile colon. Presentations include abdominal pain, distension, and total constipation. Plain abdominal radiographs are usually diagnostic, revealing a large loop of distended colon with a coffee bean shape and its convexity pointing to the upper abdomen. Barium enema will show distal obstruction, with some twisting referred to as a bird beak, but is rarely indicated.

ii. Once the diagnosis is made, treatment must be prompt to prevent colonic injury. Distal decompression is accomplished by several methods, usually using a rigid or flexible sigmoidoscope to pass a rectal tube through the anus under direct visualization. The procedure, if successful, allows rapid colonic decompression with explosive release of flatus and fecal contents. Emergency surgery is indicated when tube decompression fails to alleviate symptoms or when signs of peritonitis, ischemia, or perforation are present. Delayed recurrence of sigmoid volvulus occurs in at least two-thirds, so elective surgical resection of redundant colon is frequently indicated.

116 A 27-year-old female had a total thyroidectomy 3 days ago and presented with complaints of intermittent severe cramps in her upper and lower extremities.
i. What does this photograph suggest is the problem here (**116**)?
ii. How should she be managed?

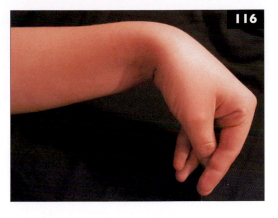

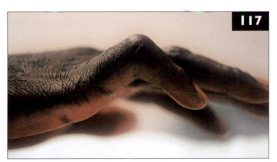

117 A 35-year-old female lacerated her fifth finger on a broken glass while washing dishes 2 days ago. She was unable to straighten her finger (**117**).
i. Can you explain what is going on?
ii. How should she be managed?

116 i. Post-thyroidectomy hypocalcemia develops in up to 25% of people after total thyroidectomy and is symptomatic in about 10%. It may be transient or permanent. It is usually mild, but occasionally can be life threatening. Thyroid carcinoma, hyperthyroidism, and total thyroidectomy are the main predisposing factors for parathyroid hypofunction after this surgery, leading to post-thyroidectomy hypocalcemia. Patients present with muscle cramps, including carpopedal spasms (as seen here), as well as circumoral and extremity numbness, seizures, prolonged QT interval on ECG, and cardiac pump dysfunction. Chvostek's sign (twitching of ipsilateral circumoral muscles with tapping over facial nerve near the ear) and Trousseau's sign (carpopedal spasm provoked by ischemia from BP cuff inflated above systolic pressure for up to 3 minutes) are common physical examination signs. Hyperventilation may also exacerbate symptoms by inducing alkalosis.

ii. Measure serum electrolytes, calcium (including ionized calcium if available), and magnesium to confirm symptom etiology. IV calcium gluconate should be given slowly, unless cardiac arrest occurs due to hypocalcemia. Coexisting hypomagnesemia is common and should also be treated. Oral calcium preparations may achieve adequate calcium repletion, but vitamin D supplements are often needed. Post-thyroidectomy hypocalcemia tends to resolve over time and usually does not require long-term therapy.

117 i. This is an acute traumatic boutonnière deformity, also called a forked finger, with flexion at the proximal interphalangeal joint while the distal one is extended. It is due to rupture of the dorsally located central slip of the extensor mechanism, which allows the lateral bands to migrate volarly. Here the etiology is traumatic due to direct central slip laceration, but forced flexion of the extended proximal interphalangeal joint or its dislocation can also tear the central slip. Nontraumatic causes include rheumatoid arthritis and other arthritides, full-thickness burns, and infections. Acute traumatic boutonnière deformity will present with this finger posture, but will allow and maintain passive extension. Over time, lateral band contractures will not allow extension.

ii. This deformity will require surgical intervention. Cases with volar proximal interphalangeal dislocation that cannot be reduced and those with displaced avulsions of the dorsal base of the middle phalanx will also need surgery. Splinting in extension is indicated for traumatic boutonnière deformity to reduce lateral band contracture. Surgical reconstruction is complex and requires an experienced orthopedic or hand surgeon.

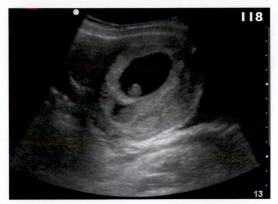

118 A 26-year-old female presented with lower abdominal pain and vaginal bleeding. She thought her last menstrual period ended about 6 weeks ago.
i. What does this ultrasound image show (118)?
ii. What should you tell her about this clinical situation?

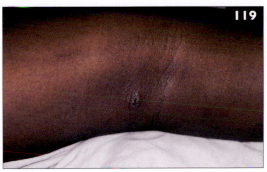

119 A 21-year-old female presented with multiple sore joints and several lesions, like the one shown on her skin (119), which had developed over the past few days.
i. What should we be thinking of here?
ii. How should she be evaluated and treated?

118 i. Significant first-trimester vaginal bleeding occurs in one in four pregnancies, and about half will miscarry. The ultrasound image shows intrauterine pregnancy with subchorionic hemorrhage (bleeding between uterus and placenta) that is partially clotted. Early pregnancy failure can be diagnosed by absence of visible yolk sac with a gestational sac diameter of 13 mm or more, absence of visible embryo if the gestational sac is 20 mm or more in diameter, or absence of cardiac motion with an embryo measuring 5 mm or more in maximum length. Documentation of intrauterine pregnancy virtually excludes an ectopic pregnancy. Heterotopic pregnancy (intrauterine and concomitant ectopic) occurs in 1 in 4,000 to 1 in 5,000 pregnancies (although much more frequent with in-vitro fertilization). Approximately 20% of women with first trimester bleeding have subchorionic hemorrhage.

ii. Tell her she has an intrauterine pregnancy. The embryo is clearly much larger than 5 mm, so viability can be determined by presence or absence of cardiac activity. In first trimester vaginal bleeding, subchorionic hemorrhage of small volume does not significantly correlate with pregnancy failure.

119 i. This is disseminated gonococcal infection, which has two phases: an early bacteremic phase with arthralgias, tenosynovitis, and dermatitis, and a late phase represented by septic arthritis. Endocarditis, osteomyelitis, meningitis, and sepsis are rare complications. Menstruating and pregnant women, as well as those with immunodeficiency or complement deficiencies, are at particular risk. *Neisseria gonorrhea* usually spreads from the cervix, urethra, rectum, or pharynx and disseminates via the bloodstream. The bacteremic phase occurs during the first 2–3 days of gonococcemia, with concomitant fever and other constitutional symptoms. Classic skin lesions in disseminated gonococcal infection are hemorrhagic pustules on the extremities.

ii. Diagnosis is made by culture, PCR, or other serologic tests from the cervix, urethra, rectum, and pharynx. Aspiration of affected joints may be useful. Treatment for both gonococcal infection and presumed coinfection with *Chlamydia trachomatis* is recommended. A third-generation cephalosporin (e.g. ceftriaxone) and doxycycline (not in pregnancy) or azithromycin is recommended.

120 A 48-year-old female had 1 year of increasing dyspnea, with abdominal and lower extremity swelling. She also described frequent diarrhea along with early satiety. She smoked one pack of cigarettes daily, but had no known medical problems. She appeared chronically ill, with BP of 94/60 mmHg (12.5/8.0 kPa), P 104 bpm, RR 24/min, and T 37.8°C. She had a few diffuse wheezes on pulmonary examination and had a normal cardiac examination. She had a distended abdomen with a positive fluid wave, and her liver was palpable 4 cm below the right costal margin. She had pitting edema to her knees bilaterally.

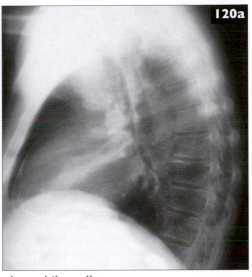

i. What does this lateral chest radiograph suggest (**120a**)?
ii. How should the patient be evaluated?
iii. What is the appropriate therapy?

121 A 37-year-old male with a history of hypertension, diabetes mellitus, and hyperlipidemia presented with this rash (**121**). He recalled a night of heavy eating and alcohol use.

i. What is this rash, and what caused it?
ii. What treatment is indicated?

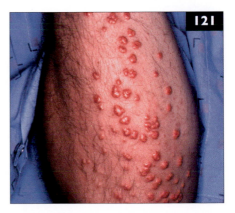

120 i. A thin layer of pericardial calcification (seen in CT image **120b**, arrows), usually due to prior infectious pericarditis or trauma. It is occasionally seen with systemic lupus erythematosus, rheumatic heart disease, hemopericardium, or uremia. Calcified pericardium is strongly associated with constrictive pericarditis, where a thickened, fibrotic pericardium impedes diastolic filling. Symptoms often progress slowly over months to years,

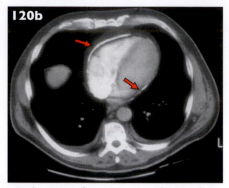

with delayed diagnosis common. Dyspnea is the most frequent complaint, along with fatigue, lower extremity edema, abdominal distension, nausea, diarrhea, and early satiety. Jugular venous distension is a constant, with sinus tachycardia and muffled heart sounds common.

ii. Symptoms and examination findings are nonspecific, making clinical diagnosis difficult. Constrictive pericarditis is not associated with classic ECG findings of acute pericarditis. Chest radiography is not usually diagnostic, although these somewhat rare pericardial calcifications are suggestive. No echocardiographic findings are pathognomonic, but Doppler and other techniques can give suggestive hemodynamic information. MRI best evaluates pericardial thickness and calcifications, but does not prove constriction is present. CT is less helpful, unless special techniques are used. Usually, the diagnosis of constrictive pericarditis is based on a combination of tests.

iii. Treat the underlying cause. Complete pericardiectomy is definitive and may be curative, with modern surgical mortalities of 5–6%.

121 i. Eruptive xanthomas, red–yellow fat-laden papules on an erythematous base that appear in groups on the buttocks, extensor surfaces of extremities, and shoulders. They may be associated with itching or pain. Eruptive xanthomas occur in the presence of chylomicronemia and hypertriglyceridemia. They are seen with type I, type V, and, rarely, type IV hyperlipoproteinemias. Eruptive xanthomas may be seen with uncontrolled diabetes mellitus, hypothyroidism, nephrotic syndrome, and with excessive estrogen, glucocorticoid, alcohol, or retinoid use.

ii. Treatment usually consists of dietary restrictions and appropriate medications for hyperlipidemia. Managing contributing factors is important.

122 A 33-year-old male had several days of sudden, lightning-fast, electrical shocks that shot into his arms, back, and legs with neck flexion. He also stated he felt weak and unsteady while walking. He admitted to abuse of alcohol, cocaine, and marijuana, as well as inhaling gas from whipping cream cans. His neurologic examination was completely normal, and cervical spine radiographs with flexion and extension views were perfect.
i. Is there a name for the complaint the patient describes?
ii. Is there a real medical problem here?

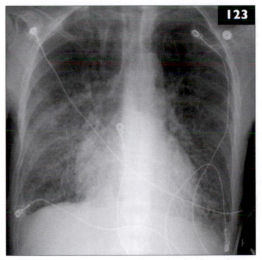

123 A previously healthy 28-year-old female had a fever for 2 days with nonproductive cough and increased fatigue. She presented after passing out at home and was confused. BP was 72/48 mmHg (9.6/6.4 kPa), P 148 bpm, RR 32/min, and T 39.4°C.
i. What does the clinical picture and this chest radiograph suggest (**123**)?
ii. How should she be treated?

122 i. Lhermitte's sign is an electrical sensation running down the back and into the limbs from involvement of the posterior columns, elicited by neck flexion or extension. Although a classic sign in multiple sclerosis, it is also reported with trauma, radiation myelopathy, spinal cord compression (e.g. disk herniation), systemic lupus erythematosus, Behcet's disease, high-dose chemotherapy, and B_{12} deficiency. Interestingly, Lhermitte's sign (really a symptom, a subjective complaint with no objective physical findings) has been reported in dental literature among nitrous oxide abusers.

ii. Want to guess what gas he was inhaling from those whipping cream cans? Yes, nitrous oxide. Nitrous oxide inactivates vitamin B_{12} (cyanocobalamin) by converting cobalt from its monovalent to divalent form, thus interrupting its coenzyme effect on methionine synthase. Prolonged nitrous oxide use leads to subacute combined degeneration of the spinal cord with sensory neuropathy, myelopathy, and encephalopathy. Chronic nitrous oxide recreational abusers may have normal blood levels of B_{12}, but it is functionally deficient. Recovery is dependent on discontinuing nitrous oxide exposure (maybe skip the other drugs too) and multiple high doses of unoxidized B_{12}. Recovery is often incomplete.

123 i. If we stop at diagnosis of pneumonia, we have missed the full picture. This is severe sepsis with septic shock. Sepsis is characterized by an entire body inflammatory condition (systemic inflammatory response syndrome) in the setting of known or suspected infection. Severe sepsis occurs when sepsis leads to tissue hypoperfusion with organ dysfunction, lactic acidosis, altered mental status, and death. Septic shock is severe sepsis with refractory arterial hypotension. Sepsis is more common in elderly, immunocompromised, and critically ill patients, but does occur in previously healthy individuals. Pneumonia as well as urinary tract, bowel, and wound infections are common sources of bacteremia related to sepsis.

ii. Broad-spectrum antibiotic coverage (as well as antiviral agents if, for example, novel H1N1 could be the infecting organism, as it was here) coupled with aggressive volume resuscitation and judicious vasopressor therapy is necessary to combat this deadly illness. Early goal-directed therapy is a protocolized, stepwise approach to optimize intravascular volume, mixed-venous oxygen saturation, hemoglobin level, and vasopressor use. It has been shown to reduce mortality in severe sepsis. Although true adrenal insufficiency and tissue resistance to corticosteroids occurs occasionally with sepsis, it should be suspected and treated in patients who respond poorly to resuscitation with fluids and vasopressors. Early drainage of purulent fluid and debridement of necrotic tissue is necessary. Drotrecogin alfa (activated protein C) is ineffective and no longer used in severe sepsis.

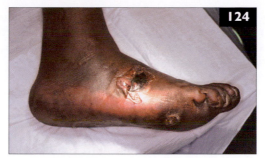

124 A 55-year-old male with diabetes mellitus presented with 2 days of increasing pain in his right foot after a minor abrasion from trauma (124). He had fever of 38.2°C, a malodorous wound with subcutaneous crepitus, and leg swelling with tenderness up to his knee. Blood glucose was 24 mmol/l (435 mg/dl).
i. What is the most important diagnosis to be considered?
ii. How is this managed?

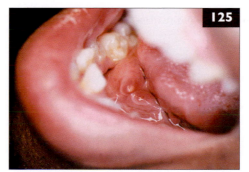

125 A 52-year-old male presented with swelling in his right submandibular region and this examination finding (125).
i. What is the diagnosis, and what caused it?
ii. How should it be treated?

124 i. Necrotizing fasciitis is a rare, life-threatening, soft tissue infection that rapidly spreads through fascial planes, causing necrosis and sepsis. Infection often follows trauma, but initiating events may be as simple as a needlestick or abrasion. Quick diagnosis is critical, as necrotizing fasciitis is rapidly fatal unless promptly recognized and aggressively managed. Often mistaken for a more benign infection, the most important factor influencing mortality is time to surgical debridement. It is more common in compromised patients, including HIV, diabetes mellitus, malignancy, neutropenia, vascular insufficiency, organ transplantation, and others on immunosuppressive therapy. Most cases involve anaerobic bacteria mixed with aerobic, gram-positive organisms. Typically, infection begins with erythema and skin discoloration, often with bullae. Infection spreads rapidly and usually causes marked discomfort. Local crepitus due to tracking subcutaneous air occurs in over half. Patients with necrotizing fasciitis may look surprisingly well, and clinical findings may be subtle. Courage to diagnose it early saves lives. A CBC along with blood and tissue cultures are indicated. Radiographs may show subcutaneous gas in fascial planes. CT and MRI improve detection in difficult cases, but may delay diagnosis or be relatively normal early.

ii. Aggressive fluid resuscitation and broad-spectrum antibiotics are important. Immediate surgical debridement of all nonviable tissue must be carried out. Repeated debridement is often needed. Hyperbaric oxygen therapy may be helpful, but has not been rigorously studied in this setting.

125 i. Sialolithiasis, with a stone visible in the distal submandibular (Wharton's) duct. Salivary duct stones are frequently idiopathic, but chronic gland infection, dehydration, certain medications (e.g. phenothiazines), and hypercalcemia predispose. Stones are usually in submandibular gland ducts, but occasionally in the parotid ducts. Patients present with swelling of the involved gland that is often painless. It is exacerbated by saliva production, as during meals. A palpable lump as well as tenderness in the gland or its duct may be noted. Complications include secondary gland infection, or sialoadenitis, often caused by *Streptococcus* and/or *Staphylococcus* species. Diagnosis of sialolithiasis is usually made by typical history and physical examination. Occasionally, sialoliths are visible on clinical examination, as here. About 80% of salivary gland calculi are visible on radiographs, and ultrasound or sialogram may be useful in difficult cases.

ii. Treatment involves increasing saliva production with sour and/or bitter food (e.g. lemon drops), which may cause spontaneous stone expulsion. Manual removal is sometimes successful, often made easier using local anesthesia. Surgical therapy may be necessary, sometimes as simple as a small duct incision, but occasionally requiring more aggressive intervention up to gland removal. Antistaphylococcal antibiotic therapy may be necessary if sialoadenitis is thought to be bacterial.

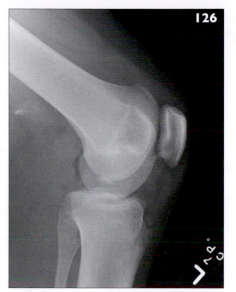

126 A 19-year-old male sustained a traumatic laceration near his left knee.
i. What does this radiograph demonstrate (126)?
ii. How should this problem be managed?

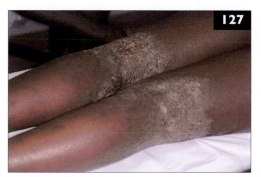

127 A 47-year-old female presented with a severely itchy rash on her arms and legs
(127).
i. What is the likely problem?
ii. How is it most effectively treated?

126 i. The presence of air in the joint space makes diagnosis of an open knee laceration simple here. Usually (particularly without joint air) it is fairly difficult to determine whether a wound near an articulation has penetrated the joint capsule. Local exploration may be misleading. Injecting up to 200 ml of sterile fluid into the knee joint space distant from the laceration, with or without methylene blue dye, and looking for extravasation into the wound, will confirm an open joint. Frequently, capsular penetration is present even without extravasation, so orthopedic consultation is appropriate in all suspected open joint wounds.

ii. Open joints are at high risk of contamination with bacteria and foreign materials. Exploration and irrigation is the standard of care, with broad-spectrum antibiotic therapy. Do not forget tetanus prophylaxis.

127 i. Eczema is a general term for many inflammatory, relapsing, pruritic, and noncontagious skin diseases. Its most common form is atopic dermatitis, and many use these terms interchangeably. Eczematous skin reacts abnormally to irritants, certain foods, and allergens. Stress or fatigue correlates with exacerbations. Eczema is associated with asthma and rhinitis. Genetic factors are important. Atopic dermatitis prevalence is up to 10–30% in children and 2–10% in adults, being more common in developed countries. Half of infant eczema resolves by age 3 years. Persistent itching is the predominant symptom, with intermittent flares and remissions. Early lesions are erythematous and exudative, but may become scaly, crusted, and lichenified. Initially, flexor areas of the knees and elbows are affected, but eczema may involve any skin. Laboratory testing is seldom useful, although scraping to exclude tinea corporis is occasionally helpful. Allergy testing adds little. Eczema becomes vulnerable to secondary bacterial infection.

ii. Dry skin, sweating, stress, and allergen exposure increase itching and rash, so employ measures to avoid these triggers. Treat eczema by bathing with non-perfumed soaps, followed by simple moisturizers (e.g. white petrolatum). Topical corticosteroids, anti-itch lotions, and tar compounds may help. Oral antihistamines reduce itching. Short courses of oral corticosteroids can control severe exacerbations. Oral antibiotics are used for suspected secondary infection. Topical immuno-modulators (e.g. tacrolimus) are sometimes effective. Eczema is a chronic condition with a fluctuating course that requires constant diligence to manage successfully.

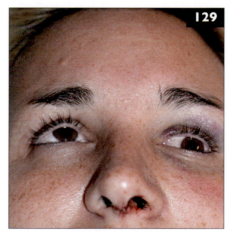

128 A 61-year-old male complained of acute pleuritic chest pain, which occurred transiently after being treated with nebulized albuterol for an exacerbation of COPD. He remained alert during and after the ECG.
i. What is the ECG diagnosis (128a)?
ii. What therapy is indicated here?

129 A 20-year-old female was punched in the left eye with a single fist blow about 4 hours ago. She developed a nosebleed and stated she had left eye pain along with double vision on looking upwards (129).
i. What do you think is the injury?
ii. How should she be managed?

128 i. The ECG is easily mis-interpreted. The casual diagnosis based on a quick glance at the ECG is torsades de pointes, an atypical form of ventricular tachy-arrhythmia associated with a prolonged QT interval. However, any ventricular rhythm at this rate should lead to symptomatic hypo-

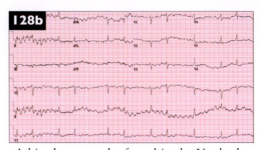

perfusion with loss of consciousness. A hint here may be found in the V_5 rhythm strip, which shows a few R waves peaking through what is actually a prominent muscle tremor artifact. This was easily recognized clinically by looking at the patient, who was shivering badly. His rhythm was actually atrial fibrillation with a slow ventricular rate. Various technical problems with ECG acquisition, such as inaccurate lead placement, lead reversal, inappropriate filter setting, and excessive signal noise, are among the many problems that may lead to inappropriate interpretation.

ii. No treatment is needed, except maybe a warm blanket and a few minutes for the catecholamine effects to resolve. A repeat ECG a few minutes later made the diagnosis more clear (**128b**).

129 i. Medial and inferior orbital walls are very fragile, perhaps teleologically so, in order to help preserve vision by allowing eye displacement in blunt trauma and thus avoiding globe rupture. Orbital wall injury is typically due to a blow from objects the same size or larger than the orbit (e.g. a fist or baseball). Most fracture the floor of the orbit. It may be asymptomatic or accompanied by periorbital bruising with swelling, diplopia, enophthalmos, and decreased sensation to the cheek and upper lip on the affected side. Evaluate the eye globe as well as the infraorbital nerve to rule out injury. Visual acuity, extraocular movements, and slit lamp studies are part of the blunt eye trauma examination. This patient had diplopia on upwards gaze, consistent with inferior rectus muscle entrapment. Radiographs may show orbital floor fracture, fluid in maxillary or ethmoid sinuses, or air in the orbit and/or periorbital area. CT may add information in some cases.

ii. Most orbital fractures require no medical intervention and may be managed as an outpatient. Antibiotics and corticosteroid use are not well studied in this setting. Patients should be advised not to blow their nose for several weeks to avoid orbital emphysema. Criteria for surgical intervention are controversial, but include diplopia and/or enophthalmos greater than 2 mm at 10–14 days as well as fracture of at least one-third of the orbital floor.

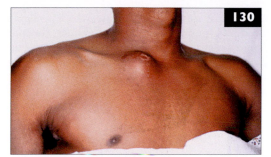

130 A 37-year-old male had an increasing swelling to his right upper chest over the past several weeks, and it began draining purulent fluid (130).
i. What is going on, and what are likely etiologies?
ii. What management is indicated?

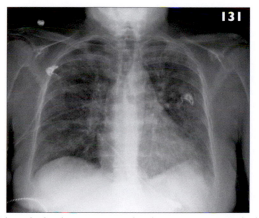

131 A 58-year-old male had COPD, multiple prior myocardial infarctions, and alcohol abuse. He presented with shortness of breath and increasing leg edema. BP was 200/104 mmHg (26.7/13.9 kPa), P 68 bpm, RR 26/min, and T 37.9°C.
i. Is this chest radiograph consistent with heart failure (131)?
ii. In equivocal presentations, are any laboratory tests confirmatory?
iii. What treatment is indicated?

130 i. This is sternoclavicular joint septic arthritis, which is rare and most frequently reported with IV drug use, trauma, infected central lines, rheumatoid arthritis, and diabetes mellitus. Here, there was no recognized predisposing cause, which appears true in about one-quarter of these cases. Patients usually present with chest and shoulder pain along with fever, sternoclavicular area swelling, and tenderness. Blood cultures are commonly positive for causative organisms, most likely *Staphylococcus aureus*, particularly in IV drug users. Arthrocentesis and biopsy may be necessary. Plain radiographs may be helpful, with CT and MRI important to assess for associated osteomyelitis (in over half of patients), chest wall or retrosternal abscess, and mediastinitis.

ii. Empiric antibiotic therapy to cover methicillin-resistant *S. aureus* as well as other potential organisms is necessary. Orthopedic surgical evaluation and management are necessary, with surgical debridement usually required.

131 i. The radiograph shows borderline cardiomegaly, alveolar edema, and cephalization of blood flow, all consistent with heart failure. Other common findings, although not seen here, include fluid in lung fissures, pleural effusions, and Kerley B lines. COPD radiographic changes may complicate recognition of heart failure.

ii. Increased chamber filling pressures stimulate ventricular wall production of brain natriuretic peptide (BNP). Assays of BNP and an inactive degradation product, N-terminal BNP (NT-BNP), are commercially available. BNP levels <100 pg/ml make heart failure unlikely, while levels >500 pg/ml are very suggestive. BNP levels are most useful if diagnosis of heart failure is unclear, and they may help monitor response to therapy.

iii. Heart failure is commonly due to systolic dysfunction, but inability of the heart to relax (lusitropy) is increasingly recognized and referred to as diastolic dysfunction. In acute heart failure with adequate BP, vasodilator therapy (e.g. nitrates) and diuretics (e.g. furosemide) remain the mainstay of therapy. Noninvasive positive pressure ventilation clearly has a role in severe cases. Beta blockers, angiotensin-converting enzyme inhibitors, angiotensin receptor blockers, and aldosterone antagonists all have an additional role in more chronic management. Cardiac glycosides (e.g. digoxin) are usually reserved for heart failure with rapid atrial flutter or fibrillation.

132 A 27-year-old male schoolteacher presented with fever, itchy rash of 1-day duration, and a bad cough. It should be noted that his wife had systemic lupus erythematosus and was on multiple medications for that disease.

i. What is the diagnosis (**132**)?

ii. What complications must be considered?

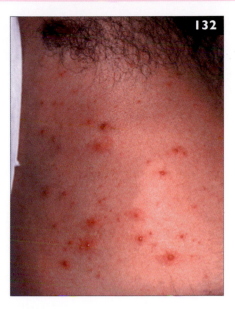

133 A 38-year-old previously healthy male presented with a week of gradually increasing right lower abdominal pain, with anorexia but no vomiting or diarrhea. BP was 138/76 mmHg (18.4/10.1 kPa) with P 90 bpm, RR 18/min, and T 37.9°C. Abdominal examination showed right lower quadrant tenderness with focal peritoneal signs. Hemoglobin was 95 g/l (9.5 g/dl), WBC count 1.8×10^9/l (1,800/mm³), and platelet count 54×10^9/l (54,000/mm³).

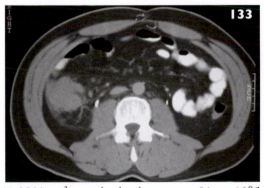

i. What does this CT scan suggest (**133**)?

ii. How should the patient be managed?

132 i. Widespread use of varicella vaccine in children has led to a dramatic decrease in incidence of chickenpox in many countries, so it is seen infrequently. This pruritic, vesicular rash in various phases of healing is clearly chickenpox.

ii. Thought is needed in managing this patient. Varicella is usually a mild, self-limiting illness. However, chickenpox has a significant incidence of lung infection in adults, which may lead to severe pneumonitis. A chest radiograph is important here. Early initiation of antiviral therapy with acyclovir, valacyclovir, or famciclovir in adult chickenpox decreases time to cutaneous healing, duration of fever, and lessens symptoms. It is most beneficial if initiated within 24 hours of rash onset. Varicella pneumonia requires IV acyclovir and aggressive in-hospital management. The patient's wife has certainly been exposed to varicella-zoster virus and is immunocompromised, both by her lupus and probably by her medical therapy. Live attenuated virus vaccination is contraindicated in immunosuppressed patients, but other vaccines, including heat-inactivated or replication-defective varicella-zoster virus, may reduce infection rate safely. She should also receive prophylactic anti-viral therapy to reduce infection risk. Close monitoring will be important for both patients.

133 i. Acute appendicitis is the most common nontraumatic abdominal surgical emergency. However, lots of things make that diagnosis suspect here. Yes, the patient has right lower abdominal pain, peritoneal signs, and inflammation in that area on CT scan. However, he has pancytopenia, lacks fever, and has a protracted presentation that just does not sound like typical appendicitis. (**Note:** The appendix does not always play by the rules, as atypical presentations are very common.) His WBC differential helped confirm the correct diagnosis, as it showed 17% blast cells. This is typhlitis, or neutropenic enterocolitis, a heterogenous gastrointestinal infection most commonly seen in chemotherapy-induced neutropenia, but also seen in primary leukemias and some other entities. The exact pathogenesis is unknown, but microbial invasion of the bowel wall leads to mucosal ulcerations, edema, transmural necrosis, and possible perforation. The thin-walled ascending colon is the most frequent site of typhlitis. Abdominal CT is the imaging modality of choice.

ii. Therapy must be individualized, with surgery reserved for perforation, diffuse peritonitis, or severe gastrointestinal bleeding. Broad-spectrum antibiotics, volume resuscitation, and, perhaps, granulocyte colony-stimulating factor are effective in many cases, but mortality rates are 30–50% for neutropenic enterocolitis. This patient was later proven to have acute myelogenous leukemia.

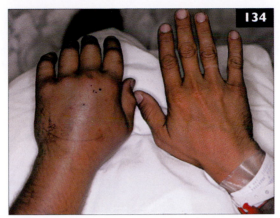

134 A 32-year-old male presented intoxicated with the complaint of just having been bitten by a snake (134).
i. What type of snake is likely to have bitten him?
ii. What therapy, if any, is required?

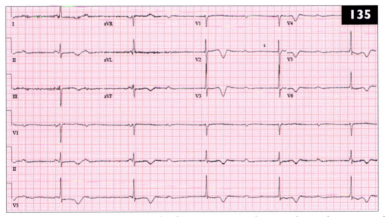

135 A 76-year-old male presented after a syncopal episode and was awake on presentation. His medications included furosemide, atenolol, diltiazem, and low-dose aspirin along with a new antibiotic given for bronchitis.
i. What does his ECG suggest is going on (135)?
ii. What therapies are indicated?

134 i. In North America, venomous snakes are of the subfamily Crotalidae (pit vipers, including rattlesnakes, cottonmouths, and copperheads) and, less commonly, the family Elapidae. Europe has mainly true vipers (Viperidae), which are generally less toxic. Vipers have hollow upper jaw fangs, which discharge mixed venom containing various enzymes including proteases, collagenases, and thrombogenic proteins. Bites tend to occur on legs or hands with visible fang marks and variable amounts of local pain, edema, and ecchymoses. Systemic symptoms include shortness of breath, nausea, and hypoperfusion with occasional syncope.

ii. Treatment decisions require recognition of fang marks and clinical evidence of envenomation, as bites often fail to inject significant venom. Laboratory tests include CBC, coagulation studies, type and crossmatch, serum electrolytes, creatine kinase, blood urea nitrogen, creatinine, and urinalysis for myoglobin. Chest radiography may reveal pulmonary edema. Compartment pressure measurement may be required. Supportive therapy includes limb immobilization and rapid transfer for immediate care. Bite incisions, mouth suctioning, ice, tourniquets, and electric shock therapy do more harm than good. Significant envenomation is characterized by severe local pain, edema distant from fang marks, and evidence of systemic toxicity by symptoms or abnormal laboratory findings. Observing progression of signs and symptoms over time dictates management. An ovine antigen binding fragment (Fab) antivenom has demonstrated efficacy and should be used for significant viper envenomations. Fasciotomy may be necessary with evidence of compartment syndrome.

135 i. The ECG shows severe bradycardia with atrioventricular dissociation and a very slow junctional escape rhythm, but no evidence of acute myocardial ischemia. Atenolol, a beta blocker, and diltiazem, a calcium channel blocker, are both possible medication-induced causes of bradycardia with hypoperfusion. In overdose, beta blockers and calcium channel blockers have similar presentations, which may be refractory to standard therapy. Both induce bradycardia and hypotension in overdose with varying degrees of heart block. It is possible that the new antibiotic decreased excretion of one or both of these medications, precipitating an increase in drug levels with resultant toxicity.

ii. Treatment for beta blocker or calcium channel blocker toxicity, or both together, is quite similar. Attention to ABC, with judicious use of IV fluids as well as careful cardiac and hemodynamic monitoring, is the first step. For beta blocker overdose, beta-agonists, glucagon, and phosphodiesterase III inhibitors (e.g. amrinone) are therapies of choice. For calcium channel blocker overdose, all of these are used as well as calcium infusions. High-dose insulin therapy with supplemental dextrose and potassium has been tried in refractory cases for both types of overdose.

136 A 24-year-old male hurt his left foot in a motor vehicle accident.
i. What does this radiograph show (**136a**)?
ii. What therapy is indicated?

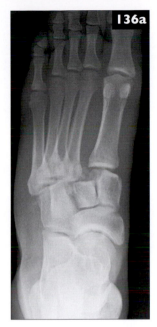

137 A 34-year-old male sustained these injuries while attempting to inhale freon from an industrial air conditioner (**137**).
i. What is the mechanism of the injury shown here?
ii. How should this airway be managed?

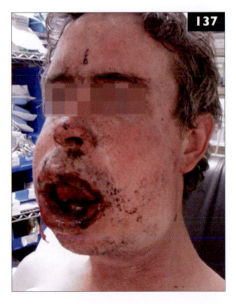

136 i. A Lisfranc fracture. The Lisfranc joint represents the articulations of five tarsometatarsal joints. The Lisfranc ligament is the stabilizing support connecting the lateral first metatarsal base to the medial side of the middle cuneiform. Injury here leads to forefoot instability. Lisfranc injuries vary from minor sprains to complete joint disruption with dislocation. This injury is rare, often missed, and most commonly due to a direct joint blow or axial loading along the metatarsals with rotational forces. In a normal radiograph, the medial and superior border of the base of the second metatarsal and middle cuneiform should align. Initial radiographs may be normal in mild sprains. Stress radiographs, CT, and MRI are helpful in difficult cases.

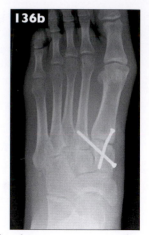

ii. Anatomically stable and nondisplaced injuries are cast for 2 weeks and then re-evaluated for stability. If stable, they have repeat casting for 4 more weeks followed by progressive ambulation in a support boot until symptoms resolve. Any instability or displacement at the Lisfranc joint requires orthopedic surgery, with various techniques for repair (136b).

137 i. This is severe oral and mucosal frostbite due to freon, a fluorinated hydrocarbon used in air conditioning systems and, sometimes, as an inhalational intoxicant. This cold injury may damage not just lips and face, but also soft palate, tongue, and lower airway. In addition, fluorinated hydrocarbons are direct cardiotoxins and may precipitate cardiac arrhythmias. They also induce hypoxia by displacing oxygen and other gases in the lung.

ii. This is a scary airway! Supplemental oxygen is very important. It is highly likely that significant respiratory tract injury is present. Definitive early management is necessary before mucosal edema makes the airway impossible to control. Fiberoptic intubation using a relatively small (e.g. 7 mm internal diameter) endotracheal tube loaded onto a flexible bronchoscope should be attempted by a competent clinician. Preparation for a surgical airway must be concurrent, with equipment and skilled personnel ready for emergency cricothyroidotomy or tracheostomy if fiberoptic techniques do not succeed or if airway obstruction occurs prior to intubation. Epinephrine and other sympathomimetics should be avoided, as they greatly increase the arrhythmia risk with halogenated hydrocarbon exposure. This patient had successful fiberoptic orotracheal intubation, but required subsequent facial reconstructive repair.

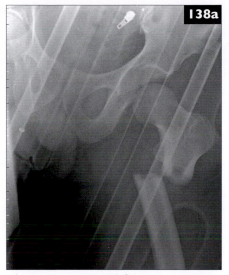

138 A 45-year-old male was a restrained front seat passenger in a motor vehicle collision and presented with severe left thigh pain. He had no other complaints, was neurovascularly intact, and had no other apparent injuries on examination.
i. What does this radiograph suggest (138a)?
ii. How should he be managed?

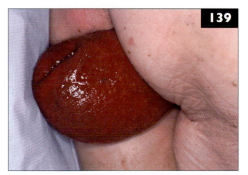

139 An elderly patient presented from a nursing home with blood in her adult diaper. On examination, this mass was found protruding from her rectum (139).
i. What is the mass, and what is the likely etiology?
ii. How is this problem managed?

138 i. There is a very obvious proximal left femur fracture. Care must be taken not to focus only on the most visible problem, which has been termed 'search satisfaction'. There is also an acetabular fracture and a hip dislocation, which a lateral film confirmed was posteriorly displaced. Prompt reduction of a hip dislocation under deep sedation or general anesthesia is felt to reduce the risk of aseptic necrosis of the hip. However, the proximal femur fracture limits options for closed hip reduction in this case and increases risk of iatrogenic injury.

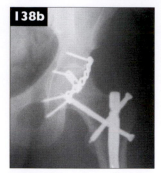

ii. Immediate orthopedic surgical consultation is appropriate, with gentle application of a lower extremity traction splint to stabilize the fracture and decrease risk of further injury. Operative intervention is necessary, and the sooner the better. Here, reduction of the hip with repair of the posterior acetabulum, along with an intramedullary rod to stabilize the femur fracture, was performed with good results (**138b**).

139 i. A full-thickness rectal prolapse, defined as entire rectal wall protusion through the anus. It is uncommon, with the true incidence unknown. Most patients (80–90%) are women, and mainly in the 4th to 7th decade of life. Young children also experience rectal prolapse. Etiology is unclear, but chronic constipation is associated. Other predisposing conditions include pregnancy, prior surgery, chronic straining during defecation, and some neurologic diseases. Certain anatomic features are common including weak anal sphincter, deep anterior pouch of Douglas, redundant rectosigmoid colon, and poor posterior rectal fixation. Initially, protrusion occurs only after bowel movement, reducing spontaneously. Progressively, it occurs more easily with events that increase intra-abdominal pressure (e.g. coughing, sneezing). Eventually, rectal prolapse may be spontaneous and difficult to reduce manually. Concomitant uterus or bladder prolapse may occur. Pain is variable, but fecal incontinence and rectal bleeding are common. Rectal prolapse is a clinical diagnosis confirmed visually, but may require straining down as if to defecate for recognition.
ii. Incarcerated rectal prolapse is rare, but reduction may be difficult. Helpful maneuvers include perianal field block with local anesthetic, sprinkling the prolapse with salt or sugar to reduce edema, and procedural sedation. Use fingers to encircle the rectal prolapse, and reduce it with constant firm pressure. Emergency surgical evaluation is necessary for failed reduction, especially if bowel ischemia is suspected. Long-term therapy includes stool softeners, bulking agents, and suppositories or enemas. Surgical treatment may be required for recurrence, with laparoscopic techniques gaining favor.

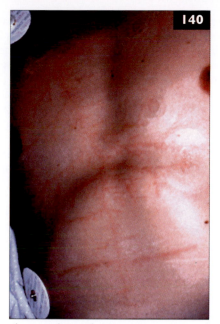

140 A 32-year-old male was brought in unconscious after being outside in a thunderstorm. He had this dermatologic finding (140).
i. What caused it?
ii. How should injuries related to this clinical entity be managed?

141 A 18-year-old female presented with lightheadedness and fatigue. She was 5-weeks postpartum and had heavy vaginal bleeding that began about 3 weeks after delivery. She reported a history of heavy menstruation since menarche at age 14 years old, which was previously improved by oral contraceptives. Hemoglobin was 68 g/l (6.8 g/dl). Pelvic ultrasound was normal. There was a family history of easy bruising and gum bleeding.
i. What do you think is going on here?
ii. Besides blood transfusion, what else might help?

140 i. This ferning pattern of skin changes is pathognomonic of lightning strike. Also called Lichtenberg figures, it looks like a fern leaf, is not a true burn, and usually resolves within 24 hours. Here, it likely explains the patients's change in alertness. Lightning is a natural atmospheric discharge causing approximate 24,000 deaths yearly worldwide. Lightning causes injury via the following six basic mechanisms: blast injury with blunt trauma; direct strike; side splash from another struck object; ground current effect when lightning hits at a distance; contact voltage from touching a struck object; and injury from an upward leader. Cardio-pulmonary arrest is the most common cause of death. CNS injuries are frequent, with altered mental status, weakness, and various neurologic injuries that may become permanent. Many other organ systems can be damaged.

ii. Resuscitation and stabilization is the goal in cardiopulmonary arrest due to lightning strike. Prolonged resuscitation efforts are appropriate, as in theory physiological processes have been paralyzed. Even patients having dysrhythmias with a typically poor prognosis (e.g. asystole) may recover completely. A thorough examination is required to exclude other injuries. ECG, creatine kinase, and troponin levels are used to evaluate for cardiac or skeletal muscle injury. Neuroimaging is indicated, along with basic supportive care.

141 i. Menorrhagia affects up to 30% of women during their reproductive years. In severe menorrhagia during adolescence, bleeding disorders are very frequent, with von Willebrand disease (vWD) the most likely. vWD is the most common inherited human coagulation abnormality and arises from a qualitative or quanti-tative deficiency of von Willebrand factor (vWF), which is required for platelet adhesion. It is actually a family of bleeding disorders of varying severity character-ized by easy bruising, frequent epistaxis, menorrhagia, and postoperative as well as postpartum bleeding. There are specific assays for vWF levels and activity. Bleeding times and platelet function analysis are also abnormal, but the partial thrombo-plastin time is variably prolonged.

ii. For minor bleeding in vWD, treatment may be unnecessary. Desmopressin is effective for modest amounts of bleeding in most, but not all, variants. Certain factor VIII concentrates rich in vWF are used for severe bleeding and, less com-monly, cryoprecipitate or fresh frozen plasma. Oral contraceptives may raise vWF levels and be helpful in menorrhagia. Aspirin and other platelet inhibitors should be avoided.

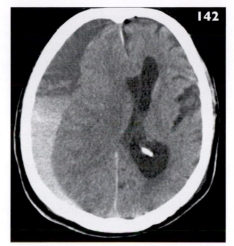

142 An intoxicated 29-year-old male presented to the emergency department hours ago and had been 'sleeping it off'. He did not seem to be awakening in a timely manner, so a brain CT was obtained.
i. What does this brain CT image show (142)?
ii. What therapy is indicated?

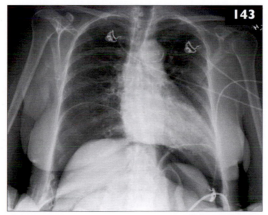

143 A 66-year-old female presented with acute abdominal pain and distension, which began 2 hours after a colonoscopy with removal of multiple polyps.
i. What does this chest radiograph demonstrate (143)?
ii. What therapy is indicated?

142 i. Significant subdural hematoma (aka subdural hemorrhage) with midline brain shift resulting from venous blood leakage. Subdural hematoma usually results from traumatic brain injury, often associated with cerebral atrophy (common in the elderly), intoxication, anticoagulant therapy, or predisposing hematologic problems (e.g. severe thrombocytopenia). In pediatric patients, subdural hematoma may be associated with nonaccidental trauma. Subdural blood is crescent shaped, as bleeding crosses suture lines. Acute bleeds are hyperdense, while subacute bleeds (5–7 days) may be isodense to brain tissue and difficult to recognize, especially if bilateral. Chronic subdural hematomas are hypodense. This CT shows a probable chronic subdural hematoma, with new acute rebleeding.

ii. Careful neurologic examination, focusing on level of consciousness, eye examination, and motor function, is mandatory. Pupillary dilation nonreactive to light on the side of subdural hematoma, or lateralizing motor weakness on the opposite side, suggests increased intracranial pressure and impending brain herniation. Treatment of subdural hematoma depends on size, rate of growth, and underlying neurologic status. Some small acute subdural hematomas may be managed non-surgically, but most require prompt neurosurgical intervention with burr hole or open craniotomy. Underlying brain injury is common. Seizure prophylaxis is recommended. Mannitol may reduce brain edema. Postoperative complications include brain edema, increased intracranial pressure, recurrent bleeding, infection, and seizures.

143 i. A large amount of intra-abdominal air not contained within the intestinal tract ('free air'). Free air, or pneumoperitoneum, is almost always very expensive, both monetarily and to one's health. In this situation, iatrogenic colonic perforation is the obvious cause. Luckily, it is a rare colonoscopy complication, occurring in about 0.1% in competent hands. Trauma, perforated diverticulitis, leaking peptic ulcer disease, and colonic malignancy are common causes of intra-abdominal free air, which requires early recognition and management. A common nonpathologic cause is residual air after peritoneal dialysis or abdominal surgery, which may persist for several days. Pneumoperitoneum may be much more subtle and is best demonstrated on upright chest radiographs. Abdominal CT may occasionally be required for evaluation and can confirm very small amounts of free air.

ii. This patient requires IV crystalloid resuscitation, broad-spectrum antibiotic coverage, and immediate surgical exploration for colonic repair.

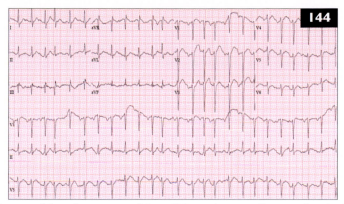

144 A 72-year-old male presented in mild respiratory distress, but he had been having recent heart racing. He had a history of COPD, for which he took several oral and inhalational medications, but did not know their names. He still smoked two packs of cigarettes a day. Cimetadine was started about 2 weeks prior for suspected gastritis. BP was 104/64 mmHg (13.9/8.5 kPa) with P 156 bpm, RR 28/min, and T 37.2°C. His P_{ox} was 94% on 2 liters/minute of oxygen by nasal cannula.
i. What does the ECG suggest (**144**)?
ii. Any thoughts about his recent palpitations?

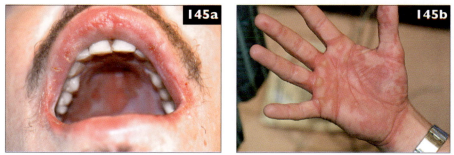

145 A 27-year-old male developed a diffuse rash, sores in his mouth, and red eyes after a few days of trimethoprim–sulfamethoxazole therapy (**145a, b**).
i. What is the diagnosis?
ii. How should the patient be treated?

144 i. The ECG shows multifocal atrial tachycardia (MAT) with a ventricular rate of about 150 bpm. MAT is an irregular arrhythmia caused by multiple competing atrial sites. This is a fairly common rhythm disturbance in COPD, but it is also seen in various pulmonary and cardiac conditions as well as in hypokalemia, hypomagnesemia, methylxanthine toxicity, and severe infection. It is rarely a serious arrhythmia, but may contribute to chest discomfort, lightheadedness, shortness of breath, and, of course, palpitations.
ii. Treatment involves correction of underlying causes, mainly hypoxia and COPD. Laboratory studies for electrolytes, hemoglobin, cardiac biomarkers, and, possibly, arterial blood gases may be ordered as clinically indicated. Remember to order a theophylline level in case the patient is on this medication. He was, and his level was toxic at 200 mmol/l (36 mg/l); therapeutic levels 56–111 mmol/l (10–20 mg/l). Multiple medical conditions and medications interfere with theophylline metabolism by the hepatic cytochrome P-450 system, including cimetidine. Theophylline has mainly gastrointestinal, cardiac, and CNS toxicities. Multidose oral activated charcoal enhances elimination of theophylline.

145 i. Erythema multiforme, an acute, self-limiting, type IV hypersensitivity reaction caused by some medications, various bacterial and viral infections, and multiple other triggers. Erythema multiforme minor involves a minimal amount of mucous membranes. Erythema multiforme major and Steven–Johnson syndrome are more aggressive forms along a continuum, damaging more skin and mucous membranes and sometimes causing life-threatening systemic illness. Classic skin findings include circular dull-red macules or urticarial plaques up to 2 cm in diameter with central clearing, often described as targetoid. Papules and vesicles occur. Lesions begin on extensor surfaces of the extremities, but can involve the entire body. Mucosal involvement occurs in 70% of erythema multiforme, usually mild with few oral lesions. In more severe disease, extensive lesions with crusting and bleeding occur.
ii. Treatment begins by withdrawal of causative medications as well as treatment of infectious and other triggers. Treatment is symptomatic with local skin care, analgesics, and antihistamines. In erythema multiforme major and Steven–Johnson syndrome, oral mouthwashes and topical 0.05% chlorohexidine baths may reduce superinfection. Systemic corticosteroids are controversial and may predispose to complications. Multiple other therapies have been attempted, without proven efficacy. In severe cases, burn unit management is helpful.

146 A 43-year-old male presented with sore feet (**146**). He was homeless, it was winter, and he had recently got his shoes and socks wet.
i. What is the problem here?
ii. What treatment issues should be considered?

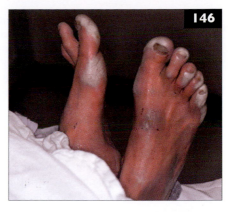

147 A 78-year-old male presented with 1 hour of severe retrosternal chest pain that had migrated to his mid-thoracic back, with associated nausea and vomiting. He had a history of hypertension and coronary artery disease. BP was 154/70 mmHg (20.5/9.3 kPa) with P 88 bpm, RR 16/min, and T 37.0°C. A chest radiograph was normal.
i. What does the ECG suggest (**147a**)?
ii. What does this CT image suggest (look closely!) (**147b**)?
iii. What treatment is indicated?

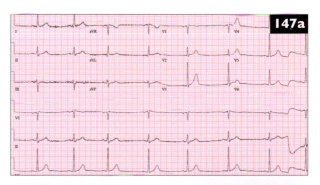

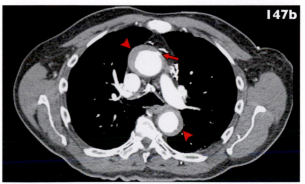

146 i. Cold exposure injuries include trench foot (or immersion foot), chilblain (or pernio), and freezing injuries such as frostnip and frostbite. This is trench foot, which is due to prolonged exposure to damp, cold conditions and is often associated with constricting footwear that limits blood flow. Feet become cold, numb, erythematous, and sometimes cyanotic with necrosis. Secondary bacterial and fungal infections may complicate the injury. The risk of cold exposure injuries is related to low temperatures, duration of exposure, wind speed, altitude, and tobacco or substance abuse. Damage is due to direct tissue injury, indirect injury from vasospasm, and vascular thrombosis.

ii. Do not rewarm frostbite until an environment exists where refreezing is unlikely. It should be done by immersion in warm water up to 42°C. Definitive surgical debridement should be delayed until there is clear definition of true necrotic tissue, which could take weeks to months. Fasciotomy or escharotomy may be necessary if circulation is compromised.

147 i. The ECG shows sinus bradycardia with a ventricular rate of about 48 bpm (with some sinus arrhythmia). What it does not show is also important, specifically no evidence of significant ST elevation or depression. Although acute coronary syndrome may present without ST-T changes, in this patient with acute chest pain migrating to the back, other diagnoses must be considered, particularly aortic dissection.

ii. The CT image (**147b**) shows extensive periaortic hematoma (arrowheads), which is always worrisome. A subtle finding is a small amount of contrast dye indenting the inner medial proximal aorta approximately 1 cm (arrow), consistent with a leaking penetrating atherosclerotic aortic ulcer. Usually occurring in elderly people with severe atherosclerosis, this is an atypical cause of aortic dissection and may be complicated by aneurysmal dilation or rupture. MRA may be a better imaging modality for penetrating atherosclerotic aortic ulcer.

iii. Surgery for penetrating atherosclerotic aortic ulcer is recommended in patients with proximal dissection, persistent pain, hemodynamic instability, distal embolization, as well as rapid increase in aortic diameter and/or rupture. This patient needs judicious volume resuscitation, appropriate blood tests including type and crossmatch, opiate pain management, antiemetic therapy, and emergency cardiothoracic surgical consultation for operative repair.

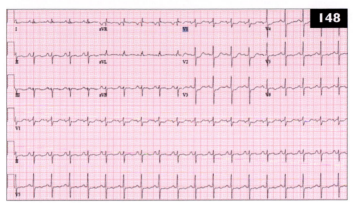

148 A 65-year-old female presented with acute chest pain of 2-hours duration. BP was 104/72 mmHg (13.9/9.6 kPa) with P 112 bpm.
i. What does her ECG suggest (148)?
ii. What treatment is indicated?

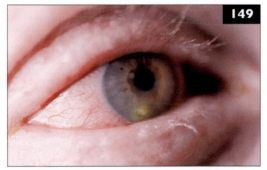

149 A 29-year-old female had 4 days of increasing redness to her left eye and now presented with pain and photophobia. Fluorescein staining of her left eye revealed these findings (149).
i. What is going on in this eye?
ii. How should this patient be managed?

151

148 i. The ECG shows sinus tachycardia with ventricular rate about 112 bpm. There are unexpectedly tall R waves in V_1–V_3, and associated ST depressions of 1–2 mm with upright T waves in those leads. (There is an unstable baseline in V_4, making interpretation difficult there.) The V_1–V_3 changes are often misinterpreted as anterior wall ischemia, but actually match criteria for acute posterior myocardial infarction. The concept of flipping the ECG over to develop a mirror image occasionally helps visualize a posterior wall myocardial infarction, as the tall R waves then appear as q waves and the ST depressions as ST elevations. Additional electrical views, including V_7–V_9 leads over the left scapula or 80 lead ECG body surface mapping techniques, can increase sensitivity for acute posterior wall myocardial infarction.

ii. Acute posterior wall myocardial infarction should be treated as an acute STEMI, with immediate revascularization by percutaneous coronary intervention (PCI) (or IV thrombolysis if PCI is not immediately available). Standard therapy for acute coronary syndrome is appropriate, including judicious crystalloid boluses for the relative hypotension and tachycardia present in this case.

149 i. The fluoroscein dye corneal uptake is the result of an inflammatory erosion. A corneal ulcer, also called ulcerative keratitis, is usually caused by infection with bacteria, viruses, fungi, or parasites. Other causes include trauma, foreign bodies, prolonged contact lens use, dry eyes (often due to inadequate eyelid closure), immunosuppression, various inflammatory disorders, severe allergies, and systemic infection. Eye pain, redness, discharge, blurred vision, and photophobia are common complaints. Although the ulcer may be visible on direct inspection, a slit lamp examination allows magnified visualization, which can be enhanced by fluorescein staining. Common bacterial agents causing corneal ulcers include *Pseudomonas aeruginosa* (particularly in contact lens users) and *Staphylococcus* species, among others. Herpes simplex and varicella-zoster cause a significant viral keratitis, often with a dendritic pattern of dye uptake.

ii. Corneal ulcers are considered a vision-threatening emergency and immediate ophthalmologic consultation is important. Corneal scarring and globe perforation are the main complications. Eye cultures may assist in management. Topical antibiotics are first-line therapy, usually alternating an aminoglycoside with a first-generation cephalosporin every 15 minutes. Some ophthalmologists employ monotherapy with a fluoroquinolone (e.g. moxifloxacin). Other agents are indicated with specific suspected infectious agents.

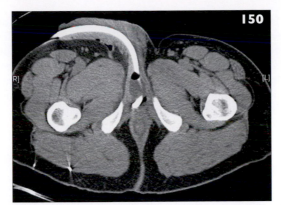

150 A 67-year-old male developed penile pain and bleeding following insertion of a urinary catheter.
i. What does this CT image suggest has happened (150), and what are the complications of this problem?
ii. How should the patient be managed?

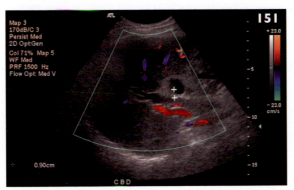

151 A 57-year-old male presented with acute abdominal pain and recurrent vomiting. He had no history of abdominal surgery.
i. What does this ultrasound image suggest (151)?
ii. What treatment is indicated?

150 i. Luckily, iatrogenic injury due to inflation of a urinary catheter balloon in the urethral lumen is a relatively rare occurrence, with exact incidence unknown. Penile and perineal pain occurs in essentially all conscious patients with urethral balloon inflation. There is also significant resistance to balloon expansion in this setting. Penile bleeding occurs in most males with iatrogenic urethral injury. Urinary outflow obstruction and late stricture formation are the main complications.

ii. Immediately remove the catheter after balloon deflation. Repeat catheterization can be attempted by an experienced physician, but blind passage should be aborted if there is any difficulty. Urologic consultation for urinary catheter placement under fluoroscopic guidance is appropriate. Endoscopic-guided techniques, as well as antegrade cystoscopy through a suprapubic cystostomy, are other methods used to place a urethral catheter as a stent. The catheter should remain in place for 1–3 weeks, and this patient will require long-term urologic follow-up.

151 i. The image shows dilation of the common bile duct over 0.6 mm, suggestive of choledocholithiasis. (If a previous cholecystectomy has been performed, common bile duct diameter may normally be up to 1 cm.) The common bile duct is recognized on this view as occupying the space between the relatively thick-walled portal vein and the hepatic artery. Its diameter, by convention, is measured from one outside wall to the inside of the opposite wall.

ii. Endoscopic retrograde cholangiopancreatography (ERCP) is the most common intervention for choledocholithiasis. Cholecystectomy with common bile duct exploration to remove a probable intraductal stone is also appropriate, and both open and laparoscopic techniques may be superior to ERCP. Ultrasound itself is fairly poor at locating stones in the common bile duct. They are well visualized by CT or MR techniques as well as intraoperative cholangiography. (**Note:** IV fluids, pain medications, and antiemetics must not be forgotten.)

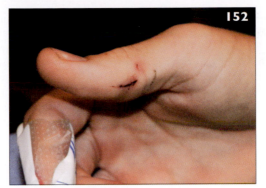

152 A 29-year-old male reported picking a bat off the ground yesterday around noon while hunting in a wooded area and being bitten on his hand. He discarded the bat and today presented with this minor, nondescript wound without erythema or any evidence of infection (**152**).
i. Is there anything to be concerned about?
ii. Is treatment necessary?

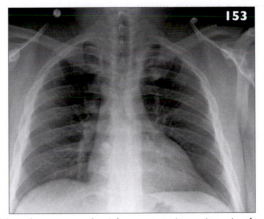

153 A 29-year-old male presented with vague epigastric pain that was worse with eating. He had a history of poorly controlled hypertension. He did not drink alcohol, smoke, or use illicit drugs. BP was 220/108 mmHg (29.3/14.4 kPa), P 80 bpm, RR 20/min, T 37.5°C, and P_{ox} 99%.
i. Is there any hint from this chest radiograph (not sure why it was ordered) (**153**)?
ii. How should the diagnosis be confirmed, and how is the condition treated?

152 i. Bats are nocturnal animals, which are not normally found during daytime and generally do not allow handling. Rabies is endemic to bats. Often, their bites are so small they go unrecognized or are mistaken for injury from a thorn or other sharp object. Rabies is a neurotropic virus that travels very slowly up peripheral nerves to the brain, causing devastating and almost uniformly fatal encephalitis. The incubation period following exposure may be weeks to months, depending on the distance from bite to brain. Although dogs are still the main reservoir for human rabies worldwide, bats, raccoons, foxes, and other saliva-producing mammals can have infectious bites.

ii. Rabies encephalitis has no effective treatment, so postexposure prophylaxis remains the only therapy for bites from potentially rabid mammals. Occasionally, the animal inflicting the bite can be recovered and observed for 7–10 days. If not ill by then, it can be declared free from rabies, obviating the need for any patient therapy. Alternatively, the animal can be sacrificed and its brain studied by PCR or viral cultures for rabies. Commonly, the assailant animal has disappeared and postexposure prophylaxis with one dose of rabies immunoglobulin and four doses of rabies vaccine over a 14 day period will be necessary.

153 i. Consider yourself brilliant if you get this one! The chest radiograph shows inferior rib notching, most obviously in the posterior 4th–8th ribs on the right (due to pressure erosion by enlarged and tortuous intercostal arteries). Coarctation of the aorta is the diagnosis, and this condition accounts for 5–10% of all congenital heart disease. The aortic narrowing is usually found just distal to the origin of the left subclavian artery. Approximately 50% of these patients have associated cardiac abnormalities. Diagnosis is frequently delayed to adulthood, particularly in the 50% with normal hearts. Severe hypertension, weak lower extremity pulses (along with decreased lower extremity BPs relative to those of upper extremity), and a continuous or late systolic murmur best heard over the posterior thoracic spine are classic physical examination findings. This man had all of these!

ii. In adults, transesophageal echocardiography, MRI, contrast CT, and conventional angiography are the main confirmatory tests. There are various surgical techniques for repair of hemodynamically significant coarctation of the aorta. Endovascular therapy with stenting is also promising, but has higher incidence of restenosis. Hypertension sometimes persists despite successful repair of coarctation.

154 A 43-year-old female sustained an inversion injury to her ankle last night while a bit intoxicated. Today, there was pain in her lateral foot.
i. What does this radiograph show (154)?
ii. How should she be treated?

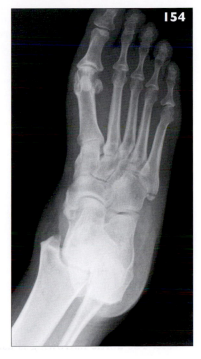

155 A 56-year-old woman had a lot of right hip pain after a minor fall, but her initial radiograph was read as normal (155a).
i. What do you think may be going on here?
ii. What other tests might better define the injury?

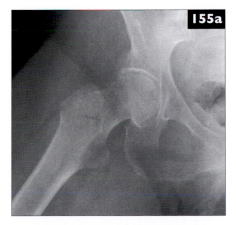

154 i. The radiograph shows a transverse avulsion fracture of the fifth metatarsal base, probably due to traction exerted by the peroneus brevis, which inserts there. The mechanism is usually foot inversion while walking forwards and is termed a dancer's or 'Pseudo-Jones' fracture. It must be distinguished from a fracture of the diaphyseal fifth metatarsal, termed a Jones fracture. While a fifth metatarsal base avulsion fracture is minor, a diaphyseal fracture has a high rate of malunion and nonunion, often requiring surgical intervention.

ii. Treatment of a fifth metatarsal base avulsion fracture is usually a hard-soled shoe or walking boot for 4–6 weeks. Surgery is occasionally needed if fragments are displaced >2 mm or if more than 30% of the joint is involved. Full recovery may take 6 months or more.

155 i. The radiograph does not show a visible fracture to the right hip. Occasionally, nondisplaced fractures are difficult to visualize and require careful attention to cortical disruption or buckling, trabecular irregularities, and areas of bony compression. Some are just not visible with plain radiographs.

ii. Other views, including lateral and oblique, may better reveal the fracture. Advanced multiple-beam equalization techniques, as well as Bucky screen film radiography, improve the resolution of standard radiographs. Digital radiography has multiple techniques to optimize resolution. Other modalities, including CT, MRI, and occasionally bone scanning, can also reveal subtle fractures. Finally, ultrasound appears to be a potential screening tool for hip fracture. In this patient, MRI confirmed an intertrochanteric fracture (**155b**, arrows).

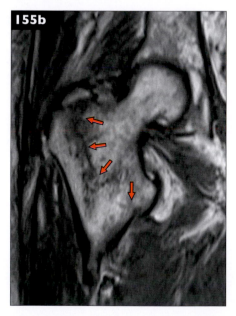

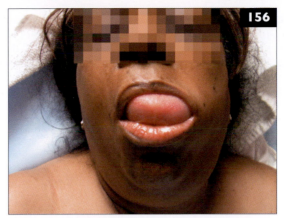

156 A 57-year-old female had several hours of progressive tongue swelling and difficulty breathing (156). She was on a new medication for hypertension, but did not know the name of the drug. She had no rash, itching, or cough.
i. What is the likely cause of this problem?
ii. How should this airway be managed?

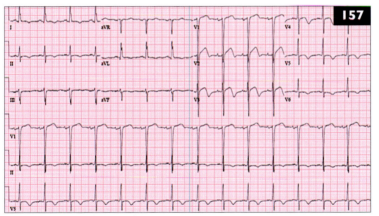

157 A 49-year-old female presented after several minutes of precordial chest pain, which had resolved prior to arrival. She had a history of hypertension, hyperlipidemia, and a habit of smoking about 20 cigarettes a day.
i. What does the ECG suggest (157)?
ii. A cardiac stress test is scheduled for this afternoon. Is this a problem?

156 i. Angiotensin-converting enzyme (ACE) inhibitor-related angioedema. This occurs in about 7 of every 1,000 people using ACE inhibitors and may develop even after years of use. ACE also degrades bradykinin and it is thought that ACE inhibition, along with some surge in bradykinin production, causes angioedema. Lips, tongue, upper airway, hands, and feet are most commonly involved. Unlike allergic angioedema, that due to an ACE inhibitor has no associated urticaria, mediator-related hypotension, or bronchospasm. It is more frequent in African-Americans and there is a genetic predisposition. ACE inhibitor-related cough also occurs in about 4% of users.

ii. Treatment should begin with discontinuation of the offending agent. Make sure patients understand they should never take any ACE inhibitor in the future. Antihistamines, corticosteroids, and epinephrine are ineffective in ACE inhibitor angioedema, but may be tried in cases where an allergic mechanism is possible. Resolution with fresh frozen plasma or C_1 esterase inhibitor concentrates by allowing degradation of accumulated bradykinin has been reported. Airway management may be difficult in severe cases, although most ACE inhibitor airway angioedema can be managed expectantly with appropriate monitoring. Fiberoptic intubation or surgical techniques are used if necessary. There is some increased risk of similar airway problems in ACE inhibitor angioedema patients who take angiotensin receptor blockers.

157 i. The findings on this ECG are important, as it demonstrates Wellens' sign: symmetrical, >2 mm deep T wave inversions in precordial leads (mostly V_1–V_4, sometimes also V_5 and V_6). Less frequently, biphasic T waves are present in the same leads (particularly V_2 and V_3, with the line slope between T waves at 60–90°). These ECG findings may remain even with resolution of chest pain. Wellens' sign is associated with critical LAD coronary artery stenosis, and in one study was present in 12% of patients with unstable angina pectoris. Wellens' syndrome includes Wellens' sign with <1 mm ST deviations, no Q waves, and minimal or no cardiac enzyme elevation.

ii. The LAD coronary artery supplies the anterior wall of both ventricles as well as the interventricular septum. Patients with Wellens' syndrome have a very high likelihood of critical LAD stenosis, and acute occlusion may lead to a large myocardial infarction with severe morbidity and mortality. Provocative testing has a high risk of cardiac arrest in Wellens' syndrome and should generally not be done. Diagnostic confirmation by cardiac catheterization, with percutaneous intervention as indicated, is the appropriate plan.

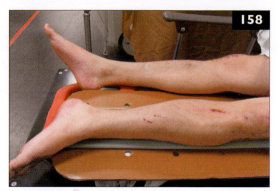

158 A 33-year-old male presented with severe left leg pain after being hit by a car (158). He did not seem to be responding to high doses of narcotic medications. A careful examination revealed no neurologic or pulse deficits.
i. What are the considerations in this case?
ii. How should the patient be evaluated?

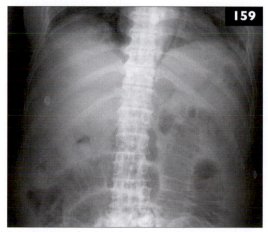

159 A 67-year-old male presented with 2 days of crampy abdominal pain, distension, and recurrent vomiting. He had a history of hypertension, diabetes mellitus, and asthma. He had no history of abdominal surgery.
i. What does this abdominal radiograph suggest (159)?
ii. What are the likely causes?

158 i. This painful fracture requires aggressive analgesia. Unrecognized compartment syndrome must be considered. Compartment syndrome occurs when perfusion pressure falls below capillary bed closing pressure (usually 30–35 mmHg [4.0–4.7 kPa]) in a closed anatomic space, with reduced tissue circulation. Long bone fracture (particularly tibial), as well as vascular injury, crush, necrotizing fasciitis, hemorrhage, rhabdomyolysis, and tight external compression (e.g. casting) are among frequent etiologies. Pain out of proportion to degree of injury is the most suggestive symptom of compartment syndrome. Loss of pulses, extremity pallor, coolness, loss of muscle function, and decreased sensation are late findings. A high index of suspicion is necessary in the appropriate clinical situation.

ii. Anything causing external limb compression must be removed. Direct compartment pressure measurement is the diagnostic modality of choice, with a Stryker pressure tonometer most commonly used. The leg has four compartments (anterior, lateral, superficial, deep posterior); all must be measured, with serial checks often necessary. Compartment perfusion depends on the difference between diastolic BP and intracompartmental pressure. Surgery is recommended when this pressure difference (the delta p) is <30 mmHg (4.0 kPa). Most surgeons also use an average compartment pressure of 30 mmHg (4.0 kPa) or more as an indication for definitive therapy, which is emergency fasciotomy. High clinical suspicion mandates emergency surgical management, particularly if compartment pressures cannot be reliably measured. Time is muscle here, with the goal of restoring tissue perfusion as soon as possible. Fracture stabilization and vascular repair should follow if necessary.

159 i. The radiograph shows multiple loops of dilated small intestine, consistent with small bowel obstruction. Mechanical obstruction must be distinguished from adynamic (also known as paralytic) ileus. Adynamic ileus may occur as a postoperative complication and it is also associated with drugs that inhibit intestinal motility (e.g. narcotics) and various metabolic disorders (e.g. hypokalemia). Mechanical obstruction has hyperactive bowel sounds early, often with borborygmi, while paralytic ileus has a silent examination.

ii. The leading causes of mechanical small bowel obstruction in developed countries are postoperative adhesions, followed by malignancy, regional enteritis, and hernias. Small bowel obstruction can involve strangulation with intestinal ischemia, which is a surgical emergency requiring prompt operative intervention. Crampy abdominal pain with nausea and vomiting is characteristic of small bowel obstruction. Fever and tachycardia tend to occur late and are often associated with strangulation, as is localized or rebound tenderness. Plain abdominal films are often suggestive, with CT of the abdomen useful to help define etiology and complications. Leukocytosis and metabolic acidosis are more suggestive of intestinal ischemia.

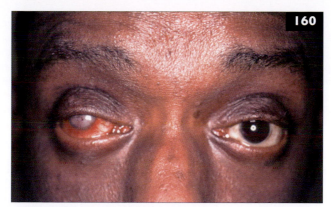

160 A 40-year-old male sustained what he thought was a severe infection to his eye several months ago and wondered if it could now be fixed (160).
i. What is the problem?
ii. Can it be fixed?

161 A 32-year-old female presented 6-days postpartum with altered mental status and a new-onset generalized seizure. BP was 184/108 mmHg (24.5/14.4 kPa) and P 126 bpm.
i. What is the preliminary diagnosis?
ii. How should she be managed?

160 i. Severe corneal neovascularization, which is usually due to an ocular insult such as chemical injury, infectious keratitis, various immunologic conditions, trauma, or prolonged contact lens use. Infectious causes include herpes simplex and zoster, measles, syphilis, or tuberculosis. A frequent cause worldwide is onchocerciasis, also known as river blindness, a parasitic disease caused by infection with the nematode *Onchocerca volvulus* (second most common cause of infectious blindness). Corneal neovascularization is thought to be secondary to hypoxic or inflammatory disruption of the corneal immune system. New blood vessels grow from the limbus into the normally avascular cornea, with a secondary inflammatory response. This may be mild and asymptomatic or become severe and threaten visual function.
ii. The primary treatment is elimination of the underlying cause. Topical and sub-conjunctival corticosteroids may be helpful. Bevacizumab combined with superficial keratectomy may be helpful for ocular surface neovascularization. Laser zapping of the neovascularization may help in some cases. In this case, corneal transplantation is the only solution, but there is almost a two-fold risk of corneal transplant failure with severe neovascularization.

161 i. Eclampsia is defined as new-onset seizures or unexplained coma during late pregnancy or in the early postpartum period. Usually, these patients have prior pre-eclampsia with the triad of pregnancy-related hypertension, proteinuria, and peripheral edema. Pre-eclampsia and eclampsia typically occur in the third trimester or early postpartum period, but are reported up to 23 days after delivery. Definitive pathophysiology is unknown, but there are derangements in multiple organs including the hematologic, renal, hepatic, cardiovascular, and central nervous systems. Incidence of eclampsia is higher in developing countries and twice as frequent in blacks. It presents with headache, hyperreflexia, proteinuria, edema, visual disturbances, and upper abdominal pain, but seizure may be the first manifestation of eclampsia. Work-up includes CBC, urinalysis, serum electrolytes including calcium and magnesium, liver function tests, and glucose. Neuroimaging may be necessary to exclude intracranial hemorrhage, cerebral venous thrombosis, or other CNS disorders, particularly in patients not responding to standard therapy.
ii. Eclampsia is life threatening. Employ left lateral decubitus position to reduce inferior vena cava compression if the patient is still pregnant. Administer magnesium sulfate to treat and prevent subsequent seizures. Use benzodiazepines (e.g. lorazepam) for refractory seizures. Control hypertension with agents such as labetalol or hydralazine. Delivery is optimal treatment for eclampsia in pregnancy, after primary stabilization. Cesarean section should be done if not quickly stabilized or for other obstetric indications.

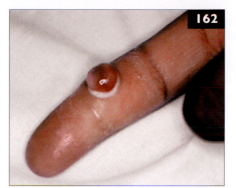

162 A 34-year-old female had a growing mass on her finger (**162**) for a couple of weeks. It developed after minor trauma.
i. What is this mass?
ii. How should it be managed?

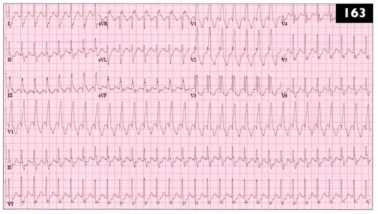

163 This ECG (**163**) is from a 73-year-old male who reported an hour of palpitations and mild shortness of breath, without any chest pain. He had two previous myocardial infarctions and had an implanted cardioverter-defibrillator. BP was 100/64 mmHg (13.3/8.5 kPa) and P 176 bpm.
i. What is this rhythm?
ii. Why has his cardioverter-defibrillator not fired to resolve this arrhythmia?
iii. How should he be treated?

162 i. A pyogenic granuloma, a relatively common hypervascular skin growth. It presents as a red oozing nodule that frequently bleeds. It often develops after minor injury and grows over a few weeks to an average size of 1 centimeter or more. Pyogenic granuloma is most common in children, pregnant women, and those taking certain medications (e.g. oral contraceptives). They usually occur on the head, neck, upper trunk, hands, and feet. Pyogenic granulomas are always benign, but may mimic cancerous growth. Biopsy may be necessary in questionable cases.

ii. Most pyogenic granulomas can be removed under local anesthesia with a scalpel or curette, using local cautery. Bleeding on removal is common, should be anticipated, and can be controlled using silver nitrate, phenol, or podophyllin. Recurrence happens in up to 50%. The highest cure rate is obtained with full-thickness surgical excision. Laser therapy has also been used with some success.

163 i. This wide-complex, regular tachycardia has a rate of about 176 bpm. With previous myocardial infarction, a rapid, wide-complex rhythm is ventricular tachycardia in about 97% of cases. The main differential diagnosis is supraventricular tachycardia with aberrancy. Several different schemes have been described to distinguish ventricular from supraventricular tachycardia with abberancy, but they are somewhat complex. If uncertain, assume ventricular tachycardia.

ii. The cardioverter-defibrillator is expected to shock this rhythm. There are various reasons for failure, including battery exhaustion or other mechanical problems, but programing issues are common. To protect from shocking sinus tachycardia or other nonthreatening cardiac rhythms, there is a minimum programable rate at which shocks will be delivered. In this case, his defibrillator's minimum firing rate was set at 188 bpm. (Oops!)

iii. Ventricular tachycardia is not always an immediate emergency. If perfusion is adequate, significant heart failure does not exist, and no evidence of acute myocardial ischemia is present, the rhythm may be treated with IV medications or cardioversion. Amiodarone is favored over lidocaine, with procainamide a third-line agent because of its tendency to exacerbate heart failure. If hypoperfusion, myocardial ischemia, or decreased consciousness occurs, immediate cardioversion using 100–200 joule biphasic shocks should resolve the arrhythmia. Interestingly, in this case the rhythm resolved after a technician programed a device shock. It was also reprogramed to respond to tachycardia at a lower rate.

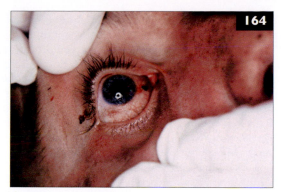

164 A 33-year-old male was found unconscious in a garage. It was initially unclear what happened to him. On arrival, he was restless and confused. BP was 190/100 mmHg (25.3/13.3 kPa) with P 60 bpm.
i. What does this picture suggest (**164**)?
ii. What test is most important here?

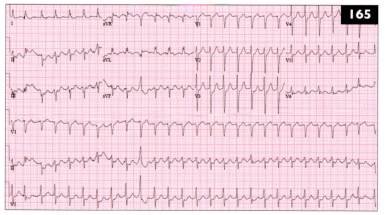

165 A 34-year-old male presented with new-onset palpitations. He had a history of previous heart rhythm problems. He was on no medications and was alert with a normal BP.
i. What is this rhythm (**165**)?
ii. How should this be managed?

164 i. The patient has a dilated pupil with conjunctival and facial petechiae. Certainly, many things are in the differential diagnosis, but one concern is traumatic asphyxia (aka Perthes syndrome). This develops secondary to sudden increased venous pressure to the head and neck, usually from a crush injury to the thorax. Prolonged hypoxia is present in this situation, and petechiae with venous hemorrhages may occur in the brain as well as everywhere above the level of the compression. It turns out this patient was pinned under an automobile that fell off a jack, and it took a significant amount of time for him to be extricated.

ii. Neuroimaging, probably initially with a CT scan to exclude significant intracranial bleeding. MRI will give more details about the extent of cerebral edema, the main brain injury with traumatic asphyxia. Evaluation for thoracic and/or abdominal injuries is also important.

165 i. A short run of paroxysmal supraventricular tachycardia (PSVT, aka supraventricular tachycardia), beginning at the 3rd beat and spontaneously resolving with the second to last beat. PSVT refers to any tachyarrhythmia requiring atrial and/or atrioventricular nodal tissue for initiation or maintenance. It is a narrow-complex rhythm unless aberrant ventricular conduction occurs. Except for atrial fibrillation, multifocal atrial tachycardia, and atrial flutter with variable block, it is a regular rhythm. Usually, PSVT refers to the subset involving the atrioventricular node, with episodic, rapid, regular tachyarrhythmias. The most common type of PSVT is atrioventricular-nodal re-entrant tachycardia (50–60%), which involves two different conduction pathways in the atrioventricular node. Most others have atrioventricular re-entrant tachycardia, involving one or more accessory or bypass pathways connecting atria and ventricles (e.g. Wolff–Parkinson–White syndrome).

ii. Transient blocking of atrioventricular nodal conduction terminates most PSVT. Try vagal maneuvers first in hemodynamically stable patients. Valsalva maneuver (bearing down by contracting abdominal muscles while holding a deep breath), carotid massage (avoid if significant risk of carotid disease), or topical ice exposure may interrupt the re-entrant circuit in up to 50%. If these fail, adenosine, an ultrashort-acting drug that blocks the atrioventricular node, terminates up to 90%. Calcium channel blockers (e.g. verapamil) and beta blockers (e.g. metoprolol) also are effective in most cases. Distinguishing PSVT with aberrant ventricular conduction from ventricular tachycardia (VT) is often difficult. Calcium channel blockers and beta blockers may be dangerous and should be avoided if VT is possible, or if a bypass pathway could be involved in wide-complex tachycardia.

166 A 48-year-old female presented with 2 hours of increasingly severe headache with nausea. She had prior minor headaches, but nothing like this. Her neurologic examination was completely normal.

i. What does this brain CT image suggest (**166a**)?

ii. What study might be more helpful?

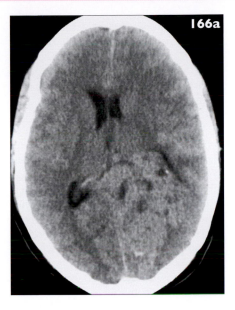

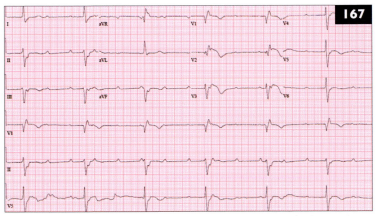

167 A 65-year-old male presented with chest and back pain of 2-hours duration. He had a history of hypertension and diabetes mellitus, with a previous coronary stent. BP was 90/60 mmHg (12.0/8.0 kPa) with P 36 bpm.

i. What does this ECG suggest (**167**)?

ii. How should he be managed?

166 i. This noncontrast CT image of the brain shows a small amount of calcification or blood in the left occipital brain, with some mass effect compressing multiple ventricles. The main differential here is malignancy or arteriovenous malformation.

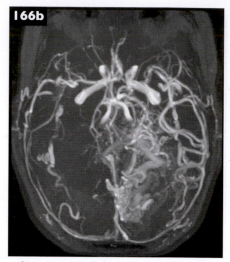

166b

ii. Using contrasted CT or MRA to define blood flow to the area will help. Here, MRA demonstrates a giant arteriovenous malformation, a huge tangle of blood vessels in the left posterior brain (**166b**). A brain arteriovenous malformation is a congenitally abnormal connection between cerebral arteries and veins, which grows over time. Many are asymptomatic, but headache, seizures, or progressive motor and/or sensory deficits may occur. Most become symptomatic at 20–40 years of age. The risk of bleeding from brain arteriovenous malformation is about 1–3% per year. This may cause sudden severe headache and various neurologic deficits depending on location, which can lead to coma and/or death. Surgical excision, stereotactic radiotherapy, endovascular embolization, or staged combinations of these procedures remain the main treatment techniques.

167 i. This patient has atrioventricular dissociation with atrial rate about 100 bpm and ventricular escape rate with right bundle branch block (RBBB) pattern at approximately 36 bpm. The subtle finding here is 1–3 mm of ST elevation in V_1–V_4, consistent with an acute anteroseptal myocardial infarction. It is important to recognize that Q waves and ST–T changes are not meaningfully affected by RBBB, so we can recognize ischemic ECG findings here.

ii. This patient needs careful bolus crystalloid infusion and referral for emergency percutaneous intervention. This is an anteroseptal myocardial infarction with complete heart block and hypotension. IV atropine may be tried to increase heart rate, but transcutaneous pacing should be applied promptly if heart rate and systemic perfusion are not immediately improved. The patient did well after prompt percutaneous treatment of an acute 100% LAD coronary artery thrombotic occlusion. He had moderate three-vessel coronary artery disease.

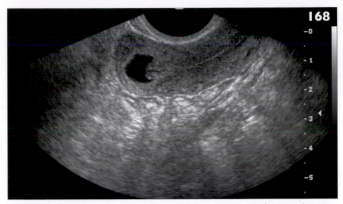

168 A 30-year-old woman developed sudden, severe abdominal pain and had a syncopal episode at home. She presented very diaphoretic with hypotension and tachycardia. Her abdomen was diffusely tender.
i. What does this ultrasound image suggest (168)?
ii. How should she be managed?

169 A 68-year-old female presented with 2 days of headaches, mild confusion, and intermittent fever. She had a history of hypertension and obesity. Hemoglobin was 86 g/l (8.6 g/dl), WBC count 9.2×10^9/l (9,200/mm^3), and platelet count 9×10^9/l (9,000/mm^3), with the blood smear showing multiple schistocytes. Serum creatinine was 0.21 mmol/l (2.4 mg/dl) with blood urea nitrogen 18.6 mmol/l (52 mg/dl).
i. What clinical diagnosis do you suspect?
ii. How should the patient be treated?

168 i. There is a gestational sac with fetal pole in an abnormal area of the uterus (other views confirmed this was the right cornu). A cornual, or interstitial, ectopic pregnancy occurs with implantation in the portion of the fallopian tube that passes through the uterine cornua. These tend to rupture later in the first trimester and hemorrhage substantially, as happened here.

ii. This patient requires aggressive volume resuscitation, along with a CBC, type and crossmatch for blood (also to confirm Rh type), and pregnancy test. Further ultrasonographic evaluation should be done to confirm intra-abdominal bleeding. Immediate gynecologic consultation is necessary, as this is a surgical emergency.

169 i. This patient has the diagnostic pentad of thrombotic thrombocytopenic purpura (TTP): neurologic symptoms (e.g. headaches, altered mental status), fever, thrombocytopenia, microangiopathic hemolytic anemia, and disorder of renal function. TTP incidence is about 5 per million per year, but more frequent in women, African-Americans, pregnancy, HIV, malignancy, use of certain medications (e.g. cyclosporine), and with bone marrow transplantation. It usually arises from antibodies inhibiting the enzyme ADAMTS13, a metalloprotease that cleaves large multimers of von Willebrand factor. If large multimers persist, they increase intravascular coagulation, causing extensive microscopic thrombosis. This leads to intravascular hemolysis with schistocyte formation as well as microvascular thrombosis, particularly affecting brain and kidneys. TTP shares similarities with hemolytic-uremic syndrome. Patients with TTP present with various symptoms related to microvascular thrombosis, which may fluctuate over time. Classic findings include confusion, headache, seizures, muscle and joint pain, easy bruising, abdominal pain, and vomiting. A CBC with smear, serum electrolytes, and renal function studies are helpful. ADAMTS13 levels are almost always low, but not readily available.

ii. Not all diagnostic criteria are usually present early, so begin therapy with clinical suspicion, thrombocytopenia, and microangiopathic hemolytic anemia. Plasmapheresis is the treatment of choice and should be initiated promptly, as TTP has very high morbidity and mortality (approximately 95% if untreated). Plasmapheresis helps 80–90%. Glucocorticoids, immunosuppressive agents (e.g. cyclophosphamide), and splenectomy have also been used. About one-third of TTP patients with remission relapse within 10 years.

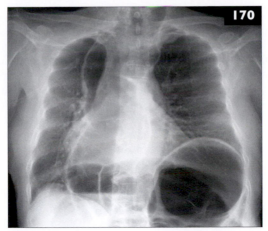

170 A 79-year-old male arrived and stated he needed some more botulinum toxin injections. You were initially puzzled until you looked at his chest radiograph (170).
i. What is the diagnosis?
ii. Why botulinum toxin, and does it work?

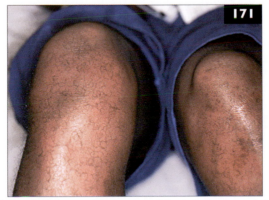

171 A 32-year-old male felt a sudden pop in his right knee and fell to the ground after jumping while playing basketball.
i. What diagnosis does this photograph suggest (171)?
ii. How is this condition treated?

170 i. Massive esophageal dilation due to achalasia, a relatively rare motility disorder of the esophagus characterized by absence of peristalsis and increased lower esophageal sphincter tone. Achalasia is associated with difficulty swallowing, regurgitation, and chest discomfort. Most cases are idiopathic, but it may be secondary to Chagas disease (a protozoan infectious disease common to South and Central America) or esophageal malignancy. Diagnosis is usually made using esophageal manometry and/or barium swallow.

ii. Changes in eating habits, along with head of bed elevation, may give symptomatic relief. Sublingual nifedipine improves outcome in up to 75% with mild to moderate disease. Proton pump inhibitors may help. Botulinum toxin injected into the lower esophageal sphincter can reduce symptoms for up to 6 months, but with high relapse rates. It is generally only used in patients who cannot tolerate surgery. Balloon dilation can be effective, but has an associated small risk of perforation. Surgical myotomy by lengthwise incision of the lower esophageal sphincter (Heller myotomy) helps up to 90% of achalasia patients and can be done laparoscopically. A fundoplication procedure, where the upper curve of the stomach is wrapped around the distal esophagus and stitched into place, is often performed concomitantly to prevent reflux.

171 i. The photograph demonstrates a high-riding right kneecap due to patellar tendon rupture, which disconnects the quadriceps extensor mechanism from the tibia. This injury tends to occur in athletes younger than 40 years old, particularly during sports that involve forceful quadriceps firing like jumping. (Older people jump less frequently!) Other associations with patellar tendon rupture include systemic lupus erythematosus, rheumatoid arthritis, patellar tendonitis, corticosteroid injections to the knee, and certain medications (e.g. fluoroquinolones). The patient usually presents unable to walk normally and cannot extend the leg. A high-riding patella and a tender, palpable defect in the patellar tendon are usually easily appreciated. Simple radiographs help to exclude fracture. MRI may better define the injury in complicated cases.

ii. Patellar tendon ruptures are usually complete and require surgical repair. Primary repair with sutures augmented by wire or other cerclage material is the technique most often described.

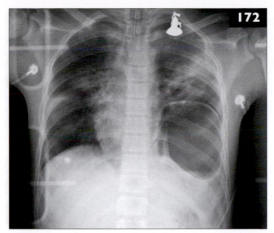

172 An 18-year-old male was a restrained front seat passenger in a high-speed motor vehicle collision. He presented with pain in his right leg due to an obvious fracture.
i. What does this radiograph suggest (172)?
ii. How should he be managed?

173 A 44-year-old male presented with indistinct lower abdominal pain of 2-days duration along with recurrent vomiting.
i. What does this CT image depict (173)?
ii. What treatment is indicated?

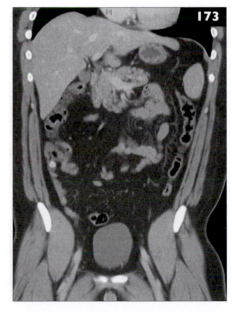

172 i. Diaphragmatic hernia (as seen here on the left) is due to both blunt and penetrating trauma, but is relatively rare. About 80–90% of blunt diaphragmatic injuries are due to motor vehicle collisions, with mechanism being sudden increased intra-abdominal pressure. Most surviving blunt diaphragmatic injuries are left-sided. However, autopsy studies suggest right-sided ruptures occur almost as frequently, have more high-risk associated injuries, and higher mortality. Blunt diaphragmatic injuries rarely occur in isolation. Pelvic fractures, spleen or liver injury, thoracic aorta tear, and concomitant head or extremity injuries are common. Penetrating trauma may cause small diaphragmatic injuries that expand over years and have delayed presentations. The chest radiograph (normal in 10–40%) is most useful by showing intestine, nasogastric tube, or other abdominal contents in the chest, an elevated hemidiaphragm, or hemothorax. Ultrasound, CT, MRI, and thoracoscopy may help in suspicious cases.

ii. Resuscitate and search for associated injuries. Decompress intestinal contents with a nasogastric tube. A carefully placed thoracostomy tube is often indicated for associated injuries, but should be inserted with caution to avoid injury to herniated abdominal contents. Surgical repair is necessary, even for small tears, as these will not heal by themselves and actually will grow over time. A trans-abdominal approach is used. Laparoscopic repair has been employed for small injuries.

173 i. Appendicitis is the most common nontraumatic surgical emergency. Evaluating abdominal pain for possible appendicitis is difficult. Historical information is usually suggestive at best. The physical examination is both nonspecific and frequently not reproducible by other examiners. Laboratory studies are not conclusive and frequently misleading. Ultrasound is very operator dependent, but appendix diameter of 6 mm or more and noncompressibility are highly suggestive of acute appendicitis. IV contrasted CT scanning (oral contrast rarely adds useful information) has radiation implications, but is more sensitive and specific than ultrasound, with the main findings being appendiceal double wall thickness greater than 6–7 mm, periappendiceal inflammation (absent in up to 20%), and appendicoliths. MRI is emerging as an alternative to CT, particularly in pregnant patients.

ii. This patient has an enlarged appendix with an appendicolith but minimal periappendiceal inflammation. He needs prompt open or laparoscopic appendectomy.

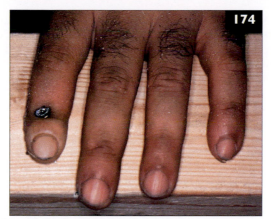

174 A 27-year-old male had a little trouble with his nail gun today (**174**).
i. How could this injury be managed?
ii. Any special considerations for removal?

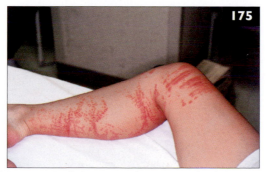

175 A 33-year-old patient had this severe burning rash after swimming in the ocean (**175**).
i. What is the likely etiology?
ii. What treatment is effective?

174 i. This was a rather dramatic entrance into the emergency department! Nail gun injuries are deep penetrating wounds, often contaminated by oil, glue, paper, clothing, or other material, including skin. Some nails are barbed and particularly difficult to remove. The most common injury site is the hand. About 25% involve bone, tendon, joint, or nerve at exploration. Radiographs are useful to recognize bone or joint involvement, but often require multiple views.

ii. The temptation to be aggressive in removing foreign bodies without adequate exploration is fraught with risk. Therefore, bedside attempts to cut off the timber and extract this nail should be discouraged. Simple nail gun injuries that have a visible exposed head, no bone, tendon, or joint involvement, and no barbs or suspected foreign bodies may be extracted under local anesthesia. Digital nerve block after careful neurovascular evaluation is often used. Local wound debridement and a short course of antibiotics seem reasonable in simple cases. This patient required operative care by a hand surgeon.

175 i. This is dermatitis caused by the sting of a Portuguese Man-of-War (aka blue bubble, blue bottle, or man-of-war), a jelly-like marine invertebrate of the family Physaliidae. These live at the ocean surface in tropical and subtropical areas around the world and are propelled by wind, current, and tides. The man-of-war has an air bladder (pneumatophore) that allows it to float on the surface, as well as long tentacles that dangle up to 50 m into the water. Each tentacle contains stinging venom-filled nematocysts used to kill small fish and shrimp. The unlucky swimmer may be stung by many nematocysts, with toxin causing severe pain and leaving whip-like red welts on the skin that last up to 3 days. The rash may progress to urticaria, hemorrhage, and/or ulceration. Severe stings may cause death due to overwhelming toxin release or an allergic reaction.

ii. Treatment begins with careful removal of residual tentacles from the skin, using personal protection to avoid getting stung. Apply salty water to affected area (not fresh water, which may increase toxin release) and then hot water (45°C), which denatures toxins and reduces pain. Vinegar is not recommended as it may worsen symptoms.

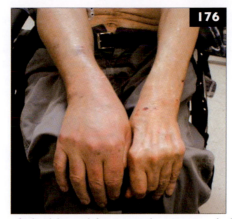

176 A 28-year-old male had been lifting weights vigorously lately in an effort to impress his new girlfriend. He presented with 2 days of increasing pain in his right upper extremity, with a sensation of local tightness (**176**). He had no medical problems and no history of substance abuse.
i. Any ideas about his problem?
ii. Does it need any further evaluation or treatment?

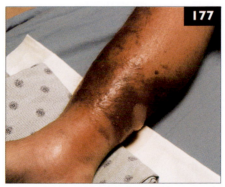

177 A 57-year-old male truck driver had 2 days of fever with rigors and painful leg swelling (**177**).
i. What is the diagnosis?
ii. How should this condition be managed?

176 i. His clinical history and examination are very suggestive of upper extremity deep venous thrombophlebitis (UEDVT), which is reported commonly in weight-lifters and other athletes. It is often termed effort thrombosis (Paget–Schroetter syndrome). UEDVT is relatively rare and is most often seen as a complication of malignancy or central venous catheters. It can also be seen in hypercoagulable states or as a complication of surgery, IV drug use, and other rare conditions.

ii. Although the clinical history and findings are suggestive, upper extremity ultrasound should be able to confirm the diagnosis, with MR or CT venography reserved for equivocal cases. Limited research on treatment of UEDVT exists, but anticoagulation remains the mainstay of therapy and is generally effective. Catheter-directed thrombolytic therapy has its advocates and it may reduce long-term complications in selected cases. Surgical decompression, venous stenting, and superior vena cava filters have occasional roles. Pulmonary embolism and post-phlebitic syndrome are main complications.

177 i. Erysipelas, an acute dermal infection caused by group A beta-hemolytic *Streptococci* or, occasionally, other species. It is more common with skin break-down, diabetes, alcoholism, fungal infections (e.g. tinea pedis), impaired lymphatic drainage (e.g. previous mastectomy), and in immunocompromised people. Erysipelas is a painful, erythematous, indurated skin infection that spreads rapidly and has a sharply demarcated raised edge. Bullae and skin necrosis occur in severe infections and lymphadenopathy is common. Fever, chills, and systemic symptoms, such as headache, nausea, and general fatigue, are common in erysipelas. The infection occurs most commonly in the extremities, but may be found on the face or elsewhere. Diagnosis is clinical by recognition of the typical well-defined rash with raised borders.

ii. Treatment is with antibiotics (e.g. penicillin or a macrolide) given orally or IV depending on the degree of illness. Secondary sepsis may occur, as may necrotizing fasciitis, so more aggressive management is sometimes necessary.

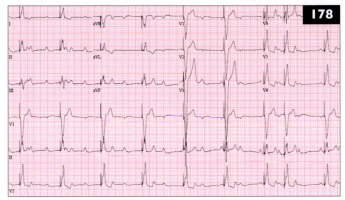

178 A 22-year-old male was born with congenital heart block and had his last dual-chamber pacemaker placed about 9 years ago. He presented with 3 days of light-headedness on standing, without chest pain, but with shortness of breath on exertion. BP was 120/70 mmHg (16.0/9.3 kPa) with P 52 bpm.
i. What does this ECG suggest (178)?
ii. What treatment is indicated?

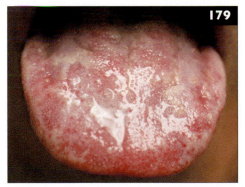

179 A 37-year-old male had 2 days of a painful tongue (179) with a fever to 39.4°C.
i. What are likely causes of this problem?
ii. How should the condition be treated?

178 i. The ECG shows a regular atrial rhythm at about 84 bpm, atrioventricular dissociation, and a ventricular paced rhythm in the low fifties. (The second to last ventricular beat may represent a conducted atrial beat.) This lack of atrial tracking and slow ventricular pacing suggests that the pacemaker is nearing the end of its battery life. Normally, the dual-chamber pacemaker would sense each atrial depolarization and have a ventricular pacing spike linked within about 0.12–0.2 seconds. As a pacemaker approaches battery exhaustion, various functions are automatically turned off to conserve power including rate-responsiveness to various stimuli and atrial tracking. Also, the rate of ventricular pacing is slow. Ventricular pacing rate will continue to decline with critical battery depletion. Battery life is dependent on many factors that determine rate of electrical use. This patient's lightheadedness and dyspnea on exertion likely are caused by failure to increase heart rate with activity.

ii. This patient requires cardiac monitoring, with transcutaneous pacing immediately available in case of complete pacemaker failure. Ask the pacemaker manufacturer technician to evaluate the pulse generator and confirm end of battery life. Prompt cardiology consultation is appropriate, as this pacemaker will require replacement.

179 i. This is glossitis, an inflammation of the tongue that causes swelling and surface changes. Glossitis may be painful or painless. It has a myriad of causes including bacterial and viral infections, irritants (e.g. spicy foods), mechanical injury (e.g. burns), certain deficiency states (e.g. iron), and dehydration, among others.

ii. The goal of glossitis treatment is inflammation reduction. Hydration and oral hygiene is important. Corticosteroids, either topically or systemically in certain situations, are often helpful. Antibiotics, antivirals, and antifungals are effective for respective infections. Nutritional therapy and irritant avoidance are appropriate.

180 A 67-year-old male developed acute headache with severe vertigo, along with recurrent vomiting. His neurologic examination revealed vertical nystagmus, but no focal motor or sensory deficits. His brain CT was normal. MRI was carried out.
i. What does this MR image suggest (180)?
ii. How should this be managed?

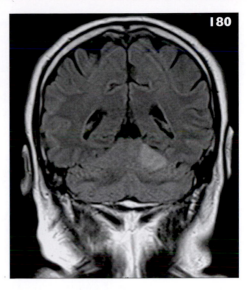

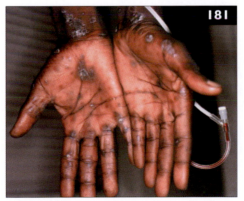

181 A 37-year-old male came for another complaint, but he happened to have this rash on his hands (181).
i. Should you shake his hand?
ii. What should you warn him about when he is treated?

180 i. This left cerebellar hyperintensity represents acute stroke. Hypertension is the main predisposing etiology, although cerebellar stroke also occurs with tumors, arteriovenous malformations, trauma, blood dyscrasias, amyloid angiopathy, sympathomimetic use, and as a complication of intracranial or spinal surgery. Cerebellar ischemic stroke may have a delayed hemorrhagic transformation. Central and larger strokes have more life-threatening complications, such as obstructing hydrocephalus and brainstem compression. Cerebellar stroke usually presents with headache of abrupt onset, associated nausea and/or vomiting, ataxia, and vertigo. There may be depressed consciousness, neck stiffness, dysarthria, nystagmus, gaze palsy, and facial weakness. Brainstem compression leads to rapid death. Brain MRI is the imaging modality of choice, with attention to location, size, and degree of compression of fourth and quadrigeminal cisterns. CT is less effective at posterior fossa imaging.

ii. Surgery remains the main therapy for large cerebellar strokes, particularly if hemorrhagic. (We might not miss some of our cerebellar hemisphere!) Ventriculostomy is appropriate for significant hydrocephalus. Craniotomy with clot evacuation is indicated for cerebellar hemorrhages >3–4 cm in diameter with altered consciousness. However, awake patients with near-normal neurologic function and a hemorrhage <3 cm in diameter, particularly if lateral and without hydrocephalus, may be candidates for careful nonoperative management by a neurosurgeon. Large, central cerebellar strokes with loss of brainstem reflexes have poor prognosis and may be managed with supportive care only. Catheter evacuation of cerebellar hemorrhages in selected patients has been described.

181 i. You should put some gloves on first. Although there are many skin manifestations of secondary syphilis, it commonly involves the palms and soles. All of these lesions are infectious and harbor active *Treponema pallidum* organisms. Secondary syphilis occurs approximately 1–6 months after primary infection. Other common symptoms at this stage include fever, headaches, weight loss, and enlarged lymph nodes. A myriad of different organ systems are involved, with many disease manifestations.

ii. Before administering any therapy, the patient should be warned about the possibility of a Jarisch–Herxheimer reaction, which occurs most commonly in secondary syphilis treated with penicillin. The reaction is characterized by abrupt fever, muscle aches, fatigue, and worsening of any mucocutaneous symptoms. The Jarisch–Herxheimer reaction is due to sudden massive spirochete lysis and usually resolves within 24 hours. It can be treated by simple antipyretics and should not be confused with an allergic reaction.

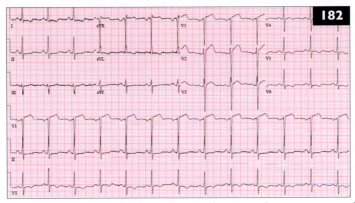

182 A 21-year-old female awoke from sleep with severe chest pressure and left arm tingling, along with nausea and diaphoresis. She was a few weeks postpartum and used oral contraceptives. She had no other medical problems and no family history of heart disease. She did not smoke or use illicit drugs. BP was 140/60 mmHg (18.7/8.0 kPa), P 80 bpm, RR 18/min, and T 37.8°C. Her troponin I level was 10.4 pg/ml (normal range <0.04 pg/ml).
i. What is going on here (**182**)?
ii. How should the patient be evaluated?

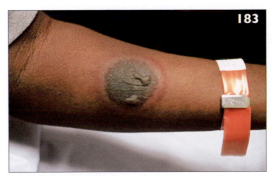

183 This 27-year-old female had a previous similar rash when she took trimethoprim–sulfamethoxazole and she was accidently given it again (**183**).
i. What do you think is going on?
ii. How should the condition be managed?

182 i. The ECG shows sinus rhythm at approximately 80 bpm, with T wave inversions in I, AVL, and V_4–V_6 and 1–2 mm of ST elevation in V_1–V_3. This looks like an anterior wall myocardial infarction. She meets STEMI criteria and has laboratory evidence of acute myocardial necrosis. But how does this happen to a 21-year-old female with no cardiac risk factors?

ii. The patient meets criteria for emergency percutaneous coronary intervention. On cardiac catheterization she was found to have extensive dissection of her LAD coronary artery with distal thrombus. She had a coronary stent placed and was then treated medically. Spontaneous coronary artery dissection is a rare but serious cause of myocardial infarction that mainly affects healthy, young females. The peripartum state and oral contraceptive use are associated with an increased incidence. Atypical presentations of acute coronary syndrome must be approached in an aggressive manner.

183 i. This is a fixed drug eruption, which describes one or more annular skin or mucosal erythematous patches that result from systemic exposure to a drug. These reactions may recur at the same site with drug re-exposure. Fixed drug eruptions vary in appearance from eczematous to bullous, as in this case. Most resolve with some degree of hyperpigmentation. Any drug, including over-the-counter medications and occasionally foods or nutritional supplements, may trigger a fixed drug eruption. Antibiotics, anticonvulsants, analgesics, sedatives, and muscle relaxants are among the main culprits. A careful history of recent medication use is the main method of identifying the causative agent. Local symptoms in fixed drug eruption include pain and itching, with systemic symptoms uncommon.

ii. Treatment requires discontinuing the offending agent, preaching avoidance in the future, and symptomatic therapy. Antihistamines and topical corticosteroids may help relieve symptoms. Provocative testing may occasionally be useful to identify the offending agent.

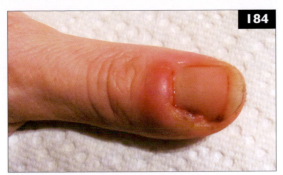

184 A 49-year-old female presented with 2 days of increasing swelling and tenderness at the base of her right thumb (**184**). She had no previous medical problems.
i. What is the diagnosis?
ii. How should this condition be managed?

185 A 31-year-old female presented complaining that the pupil of her right eye had suddenly become very big and that she was blind in that eye. She was a nurse in a large medical clinic and seemed very unconcerned about her problem. Besides a dilated right pupil unreactive to light, her neurologic examination was perfectly normal.
i. What are common causes of this condition?
ii. What evaluation is necessary?

184 i. This is a nice example of acute paronychia, a painful bacterial or fungal infection of the tissue surrounding the nail bed base. Paronychia may be acute or chronic. Acute paronychia is usually the result of some traumatic event, often self-inflicted. Acute infection occurs due to a break in the cuticle with bacterial invasion of tissue at the nail base and sometimes beneath the nail (subungual). Chronic paronychia is more of a multifactorial inflammatory reaction of the nail fold to contact irritants and allergens, often exacerbated by a fungal nail infection. Herpetic whitlow must be distinguished from paronychia because treatments are quite different.

ii. Acute paronychia treatment includes warm compresses, topical and/or oral antibiotics, and occasionally topical corticosteroids. Surgical incision and drainage is frequently necessary, particularly if associated abscess exists. Multiple surgical techniques have been described for paronychia drainage, with a digital nerve block often helpful to alleviate discomfort. In chronic paronychia, contact irritant avoidance is recommended as well as the measures mentioned above for acute paronychia. The addition of topical antifungals, as well as oral fungal therapy if onychomycosis exists, may be necessary. Rarely, partial or total nail removal may be needed for cure.

185 i. The most common causes of a unilateral dilated pupil depend on whether the patient is alert or comatose. If alert, traumatic mydriasis, retinal artery or vein occlusion, third cranial nerve compression due to a posterior communicating artery aneurysm, acute glaucoma, and mydriatic drug use are likely. In the comatose patient, intracranial mass lesions causing brain herniation are suspected.

ii. Munchausen syndrome seemed likely. Unilateral blindness is excluded by covering the unaffected eye and observing for optokinetic reflex, an involuntary eye tracking elicited by movement of an object containing a pattern of alternating black and white stripes in front of the patient. If nystagmus is present, the patient has vision in that eye. Mydriatic drug use was suspected, and several drops of 1% pilocarpine, a miotic agent, were instilled sequentually in the affected eye while observing for pupil constriction after each dose. Normally, any central cause of pupillary dilation would be rapidly overcome by this miotic's local effect, leading to a constricted pupil. The pupil remained enlarged, suggesting a potent mydriatic medication was in the affected eye. Some clinicians might still feel the need for further work-up, including neuroimaging. Here, confrontation led to admission of atropine drop use to gain attention.

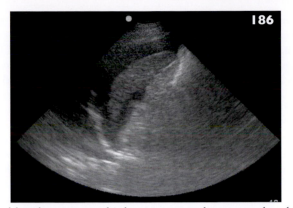

186 A 54-year-old pedestrian was hit by a car at moderate speed and thrown to the ground. He had left rib and back pain, but no other complaints. He had a history of hypertension and hyperlipidemia. BP was 90/64 mmHg (12.0/8.5 kPa) with P 124 bpm.
i. What does this ultrasound image suggest (186)?
ii. What intervention is indicated?

187 A 72-year-old male had a severe right-sided hemiplegic stroke about 10 days ago and presented from a nursing home in respiratory distress. BP was 84/60 mmHg (11.2/8.0 kPa) with P 96 bpm, RR 32/min, T 39.3°C rectally, and P_{ox} 84%.
i. What does this chest radiograph suggest (187), and what are appropriate considerations?
ii. This patient requires endotracheal intubation for airway support. Any thoughts?

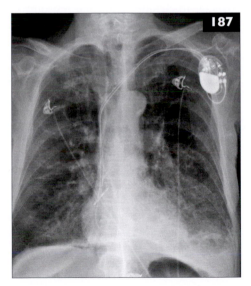

186 i. This image from a bedside FAST examination shows a large rim of hypoechoic fluid around the spleen, very suggestive of traumatic splenic injury. The spleen is the most frequently damaged organ in blunt abdominal trauma, and its vascular nature allows for rapid intra-abdominal bleeding and hemorrhagic shock. Pleural fluid is also seen, suggesting concomitant traumatic hemothorax.

ii. In the past, adult splenic injury had been managed by splenectomy, with some attempt at salvage in more minor damage. Recently, because of experience with children having similar injuries managed nonoperatively, an increasing number of adults are treated in a similar fashion. Careful hemodynamic monitoring in-hospital by experienced trauma surgeons may allow splenic salvage. Controversy exists concerning indications for surgical intervention, as significant morbidity and mortality can occur with splenic injuries. Interventional radiologists, using splenic embolization techniques, have become valuable partners in this setting. A careful evaluation for serious associated injuries is important. This patient remained hypotensive despite aggressive normal saline and packed RBC infusion and was taken to the operating room for emergency splenectomy, as well as hemothorax drainage.

187 i. There are extensive bibasilar infiltrates, left worse than right. Aspiration pneumonia secondary to stroke-related dysphagia is likely. Aspiration while supine usually involves the right lower lobe, but may be bibasilar. 'Nursing home acquired pneumonia' has the same likely pathogens as 'community acquired pneumonia', mainly *Streptococcus pneumoniae*, *Haemophilus influenzae*, and *Moraxella catarrhalis*. Recent hospitalization for acute stroke requires extending antibiotic coverage to include methicillin-resistant *Staphylococcus aureus* and *Pseudomonas*.

ii. This patient is quite hypotensive and requires aggressive volume resuscitation, if possible, prior to endotracheal intubation. (Positive-pressure ventilation may reduce cardiac preload, leading to even more severe hypoperfusion and possible cardiac arrest.) Preoxygenation is also important. As rapid sequence induction is commonly used for endotracheal intubation, select medications carefully. Barbiturates (e.g. thiopental) may cause hypotension when used as a sedative agent, while etomidate typically will not. Depolarizing neuromuscular blockers (e.g. succinylcholine) must be avoided, as they may lead to massive potassium release from muscles in recent stroke, and secondary cardiac arrest. They are contraindicated in patients with skeletal muscle myopathies, personal or family history of malignant hyperthermia, known sensitivity to the medication, or in the acute phase of injury after major burns, extensive skeletal muscle denervation, or upper motor neuron injury. This acute phase of injury probably peaks at 7–10 days after the event, but may be a consideration even 24 hours after injury. Other rare contraindications to succinylcholine exist.

188 A 23-year-old autistic male had a problem with his left ear that developed after banging his head against a wall (188). He returned after being in another emergency department yesterday.
i. What is the problem here?
ii. What should be done?

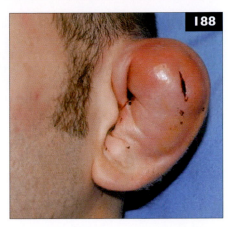

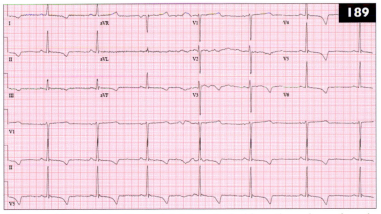

189 A 63-year-old female had been drinking alcohol heavily and was found outside unconscious in the early morning.
i. What does her ECG suggest (189)?
ii. What therapy would be most effective?

188 i. A very large traumatic auricular hematoma. It develops when shearing force is applied to the external ear, leading to separation of perichondrium from underlying cartilage and causing a subsequent blood collection. Torn perichondrial vessels may also lead to necrosis of underlying cartilage. Hematoma may stimulate new, irregular cartilage formation, leading to an auricular deformity called cauliflower or wrestler's ear. A purplish, boggy, tender anterior auricle is the typical clinical finding.

ii. Complete evacuation of acute perichondrial blood with prevention of reaccumulation is the treatment goal. Accomplish auricular numbness by injecting a ring of local anesthetic around the external ear. Multiple surgical techniques are described for drainage. Needle aspiration can be successful for small hematomas (not here!). Several incisions along anatomic auricular creases may be necessary for total hematoma evacuation. Compression of perichondrium to cartilage is necessary after clot evacuation. A simple method is packing wet cotton balls all around the auricle and using an elastic bandage to squeeze it. This allows a mold of cotton to surround the external ear as it dries. However, this autistic patient was unable to cooperate. He was taken to the operating room for hematoma evacuation and compression dressing under general anesthesia. Hematomas of several days duration also need special surgical techniques.

189 i. Besides sinus bradycardia (itself more common with low temperature), this ECG shows Osborn waves (aka hypothermic waves, prominent J waves), usually seen at temperatures less than 32°C. They may also be seen in brain injury, severe hypercalcemia, vasospastic angina, and other rare entities. The Osborn wave is a deflection with a hump or dome configuration occurring at the junction between the QRS complex and the ST segment, or J point.

ii. A prompt rectal temperature to diagnose hypothermia is probably most important here, recognizing that some measuring devices do not have appropriately low detection limits. Do not forget bedside glucose testing, as hypoglycemia is more frequent in alcohol abuse and may contribute to hypothermia. Initiate treatment with various external warming devices, after removal of wet clothing. Rapid, active rewarming is reserved for severe hypothermia (e.g. <30°C), particularly with clinical deterioration or ventricular fibrillation. If hypothermia is not the cause of the Osborn waves (it was in this patient!), neuroimaging and measurement of serum calcium are next in the evaluation.

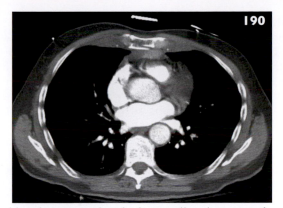

190 A 72-year-old male presented with chest wall ecchymoses after a motor vehicle collision.
i. What does this CT image suggest (**190**)?
ii. How should he be managed?

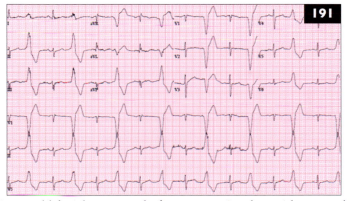

191 A 65-year-old female presented after an exercise class with severe chest pain, diaphoresis, and shortness of breath. BP was 132/72 mmHg (17.6/9.6 kPa) with P 88 bpm.
i. What does this ECG show, and what are likely causes (**191**)?
ii. What treatment is necessary?

190 i. CT reveals a sternal fracture, which occurs most commonly with blunt chest trauma from motor vehicle collision. Associated injuries are the main concern, particularly to heart and lung, as substantial force is required to fracture the sternum. Associated myocardial or pulmonary contusions are frequent, as are fractures to ribs or vertebral bodies and vascular injuries.

ii. Pain management and evaluation for associated injuries are the main issues in sternal fracture. A chest radiograph is adequate to find most sternal fractures, particularly the lateral view, which usually reveals a transverse fracture. It also screens for many associated injuries. CT reveals most other significant problems. Simple sternal fracture without serious associated injuries may be managed on an outpatient basis, with pain medication and instruction on respiratory exercises to prevent atelectasis. Observation as well as further testing may be necessary in complex cases.

191 i. This is ventricular bigeminy, a repeating pattern of a sinus beat alternating with a ventricular beat. In evaluating this ECG for ischemic changes it is important to note that sinus beats are visible in each lead without associated ST elevations or depressions. Attention to the QT interval (normal here) is also important in assessing for increased ventricular irritability. Although myocardial ischemia and other cardiac diseases are common etiologies, various electrolyte imbalances (e.g. hypokalemia), medications (e.g. digoxin), drugs (e.g. cocaine), infection, hypoxia, and other stressors may be associated with this rhythm.

ii. This rhythm in itself does not require emergency treatment as long as perfusion is adequate, as it is here. Evaluating and stabilizing the patient is important, with attention to the possibility of acute coronary syndrome. Supplemental oxygen, vascular access with IV crystalloid infusion, as well as evaluation for anemia, electrolyte imbalance, abnormal cardiac biomarkers, medication or drug toxicity, and other possible etiologies of ventricular irritability are all appropriate. Treatment of causative factors may resolve the arrhythmia. Judicious beta blockade (e.g. metoprolol) may be acceptable medical therapy if ongoing ischemia is suspected, unless there is associated cocaine or other sympathomimetic toxicity.

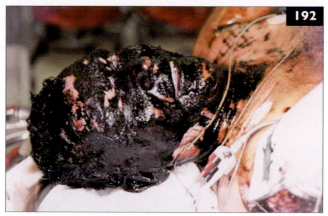

192 This unfortunate 43-year-old asphalt truck driver sustained this injury after his vehicle was overturned in a freak accident (192).
i. What does the picture show?
ii. How should he be managed?

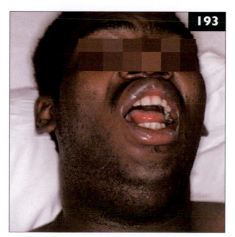

193 A 23-year-old male presented with hoarseness and severe mouth pain, with difficulty swallowing (193).
i. What condition does this patient have, and how did he get it?
ii. What interventions are useful?

192 i. Hot tar burns are relatively rare, but here the entire head, neck, and upper trunk are covered with tar.

ii. Although the appearance is startling, by now the tar has likely cooled and is no longer contributing to thermal injury. However, early after exposure, rapid local cooling is important. Attention to airway management may be necessary if there is evidence of intraoral burns. Pain control is important. Do not forget IV crystalloid volume resuscitation, as thermal burns lead to substantial fluid loss. Various nontoxic, petroleum-based solvents have been used to remove tar, including butter and mayonnaise. Surgical debridement will be necessary in this patient, with skin grafting as appropriate.

193 i. Ludwig's angina, a rapidly expanding soft tissue infection of the mouth and neck. Most cases (>90%) are polymicrobial, odontogenic molar infections spreading into sublingual and submaxillary spaces, then involving the pharyngomaxillary and retropharyngeal spaces. Combined with tongue elevation caused by sublingual swelling, this may quickly lead to airway obstruction, the primary cause of death in Ludwig's angina. Even with modern antibiotics, imaging, and surgical techniques, mortality is about 8%. Certain immunocompromised patients are predisposed to Ludwig's angina, particularly those with diabetes mellitus, HIV, or alcoholism. Diagnosis is mainly clinical. Patients present with a history of ongoing dental pain or, occasionally, recent oral trauma and/or procedures. Sublingual and neck swelling develops rapidly and there may be difficulty speaking or swallowing. Respiratory distress is present in 30% at presentation. Physical examination usually reveals firm sublingual and submandibular swelling.

ii. Appropriate airway management is the the main priority. Patients with evidence of respiratory distress should undergo immediate intubation. Surgical airway equipment should be available in case of intubation failure or if being managed without intubation. Antibiotics, often a combination of extended-spectrum penicillins or cephalosporins, along with clindamycin or metronidazole, should be given immediately. IV corticosteroids are often recommended, with efficacy not objectively studied. CT and otolaryngology consultation are appropriate. Many patients with Ludwig's angina will require surgical abscess drainage.

194 A 33-year-old female was an unrestrained passenger riding in a sport utility vehicle involved in a rollover accident. She could not feel or move her lower extremities, was unable to extend her forearms, and was weak on flexion at both elbows. She had no sensation to a level just above her breasts.
i. What is her likely injury, and at what spinal cord level?
ii. How should she be evaluated and managed?

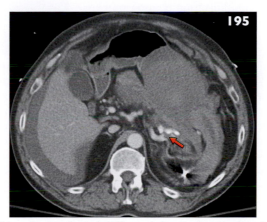

195 A 49-year-old male developed diffuse abdominal pain shortly after beginning a 2-hour flight, and collapsed while trying to get off the plane. His past medical history included hypertension and a splenectomy done 2 years ago for trauma. He had not been taking his BP medicines, or anything else for that matter. There was no history of recent trauma. He presented with diffuse abdominal pain and was confused. BP was 68/40 mmHg (9.1/5.3 kPa) and P 148 bpm. He was rapidly volume resuscitated, with appropriate blood work, including CBC as well as type and crossmatch.
i. What does this CT image suggest (**195**)?
ii. How should he be managed?

194 i. Understanding the neurologic level requires recalling anatomy lessons. C3 and C4 nerves provide sensation to upper anterior chest to just below the clavicles. Inability to extend forearms, with biceps weakness, suggests motor weakness involving the C5/6 nerve roots. This spinal cord injury is therefore at the C5/6 level and may be partial or complete. Simple radiographs can confirm cervical spine fracture, but CT more adequately defines bony injury and degree of cord impingement. MRI more clearly demonstrates the spinal cord injury (**194**, arrow).

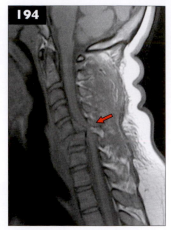

ii. Cervical spine immobilization is important for all potential traumatic spinal injuries. High cord level of sensory deficit means that pain and tenderness may fail as clues to identify underlying damage to the trunk and extremities, requiring a high index of suspicion and careful evaluation to recognize nonobvious injuries. Use appropriate imaging to recognize occult damage, including the entire spine, since multiple injuries are frequent when one is present. Ascending cord edema, ischemia, and/or hematoma may compromise phrenic nerve function (C3–C5). Carefully monitor respiratory status, with early or prophylactic endotracheal intubation, particularly if transfer is necessary. Fiberoptic endoscopic techniques may reduce cervical spine motion. Early tracheostomy may be necessary. Neurogenic shock with hypotension and bradycardia is expected. Evaluate perfusion using clinical examination, urine output, and hemodynamic monitoring. Immediate neurosurgical consultation is important, as cervical spine realignment and surgical stabilization may improve recovery in some cases. High-dose corticosteroid (e.g. methylprednisolone) use is controversial in blunt spinal cord injury and likely of limited utility here. Discuss use with the neurosurgeon.

195 i. This is an amazing image, showing a vascular blush from the splenic artery surgical stump (arrow) and a huge amount of intra-abdominal blood. This is a rare delayed postsplenectomy complication. This man is very lucky it was not a longer flight!

ii. He is in hemorrhagic shock and needs aggressive IV crystalloid, blood transfusions, and immediate surgical consultation. Although interventional radiology might be able to embolize this leaking artery in sophisticated centers, emergency laparotomy is the traditional solution for problems of this type. If he survives (he did), postoperative assessment for appropriate immunizations is important for this postsplenectomy patient.

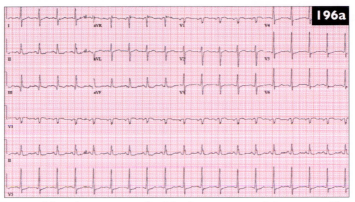

196 A 75-year-old patient presented with abrupt onset of shortness of breath after a sudden syncopal episode. He had a history of transurethral prostatectomy 4 weeks ago. BP was 92/50 mmHg (12.3/6.7 kPa), with P 116 bpm and RR 24/min.
i. What diagnosis does this ECG suggest (196a)?
ii. How should the diagnosis be confirmed?

197 A 72-year-old male presented with acute chest pain and had a syncopal episode just before arrival. BP was 84/56 mmHg (11.2/7.5 kPa) with P 76 bpm. He was noted to have a soft, early diastolic murmur in his left anterior upper chest and diminished femoral pulses.
i. What does this chest radiographic image suggest (197)?
ii. How should this diagnosis be confirmed?

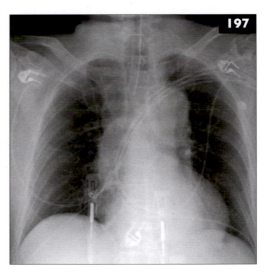

196 i. The ECG shows sinus tachycardia with a $S_1Q_3T_3$ pattern consistent with acute right heart strain, very suggestive of acute pulmonary embolism. Sinus tachycardia is the most frequent ECG abnormality in acute pulmonary embolism. In cases of massive and submassive pulmonary embolism, anterior and inferior T wave inversions are a frequently recognized ECG finding. The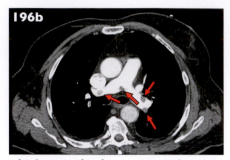
$S_1Q_3T_3$ pattern of acute heart strain is fairly specific for severe pulmonary embolism, but less frequent than previously thought.

ii. Contrasted spiral CT chest angiography is the confirmatory test of choice for pulmonary embolism (**196b**, arrows). Ventilation–perfusion lung scanning, MRA (lower sensitivity), and, rarely today, pulmonary angiography are alternative techniques. Remember that lower extremity venous Doppler studies may be done instead to confirm deep venous thrombophlebitis, which if present in this setting, makes pulmonary embolism intuitively obvious.

197 i. Widened superior mediastinum suggests acute aortic dissection. Although 8 cm is used as a top limit for superior mediastinal width, films are often supine, anterior–posterior, or poor quality, making subjective impression of increased width useful. Proximal dissection originates in the ascending aorta or aortic arch, while distal dissection begins after the left subclavian takeoff.

ii. Search for clinical evidence suggesting aortic dissection. Extremity pulse deficits occur in 50% of proximal and about 15% of distal dissection. Aortic regurgitation is common in proximal dissection. In unstable patients, transesophageal echocardiography has excellent sensitivity, much better than transthoracic studies. In patients with good perfusion, spiral CT and MRI are highly sensitive and specific. Aortography is still occasionally used. In hypoperfusion with reasonable suspicion of aortic dissection, IV fluids are indicated, with blood products and vasopressors as needed. Hypotension is a bad prognostic sign and should prompt concern about associated aortic regurgitation (as in this case), cardiac tamponade, or aortic rupture. IV narcotics have favorable hemodynamic effects and are aggressively employed, unless precluded by severe hypotension. With adequate BP, beta blocker therapy is recommended, reducing contractility, heart rate, and BP and thus limiting aortic dissection propagation. Prompt cardiothoracic surgical consultation is indicated. Time is critical, with one-third dying within 24 hours without surgical repair. Almost all acute proximal and many distal dissections need prompt surgery. Intravascular stenting has an increasing role.

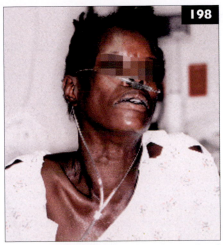

198 A 41-year-old female presented with a few days of palpitations, along with increased shortness of breath, anxiety, and confusion (**198**). She had a narrow-complex, irregular heart rhythm at 160–190 bpm and fever of 40.2°C.
i. What does this clinical picture suggest, and how should the diagnosis be confirmed?
ii. How should treatment be initiated?

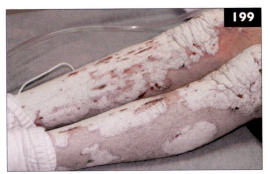

199 This unfortunate 37-year-old male had AIDS and this rash (**199**).
i. What is this condition?
ii. What management may help?

198 i. This patient has an enlarged thyroid and, in this setting, probably severe hyperthyroidism with thyroid storm, a life-threatening medical condition due to severe thyrotoxicosis. Thyroid storm is usually associated with fever, altered mental status, vomiting and/or diarrhea, weakness, and cardiac arrhythmias with heart failure. Common triggers include discontinuation of drugs used to treat hyperthyroidism, severe infection or stress with underlying hyperactive thyroid, or radioactive iodine administration. Elevated thyroid hormone levels will confirm diagnosis of thyroid storm, but this condition should be suspected and treatment begun promptly with reasonable clinical suspicion. Untreated, mortality approaches 100%.

ii. Treatment includes medications to decrease circulating thyroid hormones, blunt their effects on end organs, and reduce hormone production. Rapid beta blockade (e.g. propranolol) will control heart rate and decrease myocardial irritability, while reducing T_4 to T_3 conversion. Antithyroid compounds (e.g. propylthiouracil) block synthesis of and peripheral conversion of thyroid hormone. After initiating the above therapies, thyroid hormone release can be reduced by large doses of iodine, with the radiocontrast agent sodium ipodate preferred, as it also reduces T_4 to T_3 conversion. Patients intolerant to iodine can use lithium to block thyroid hormone release. Glucocorticoids are also important and have been shown to improve survival in thyroid storm. In addition, IV fluids, electrolyte correction, antipyretic therapy (e.g. paracetamol), and other supportive measures are important. Aspirin should be avoided, as it displaces thyroid hormone from protein-binding sites.

199 i. This is an extremely severe case of psoriasis, a chronic immune-mediated skin disease that affects 1–3% of HIV-infected patients. Psoriasis may commonly present as the first clinical manifestation of HIV, but may also be a late complication of AIDS. Paradoxically, it is a T cell-mediated skin condition.

ii. Topical therapy remains the mainstay of psoriasis treatment in HIV infection, particularly topical corticosteroids, vitamin D, and cytokine inhibitors (e.g. ustekinumab). In resistant cases, ultraviolet therapy with or without psoralens may prove helpful. Systemic therapy with cyclosporine as well as tumor necrosis factor inhibitors (e.g. etanercept) may be helpful in recalcitrant cases, with careful monitoring. Finally, effective HIV therapy may improve psoriasis in many of these patients.

200 A 54-year-old female presented with sudden onset of flashing lights and floating black spots in her right eye. She recalled no trauma.
i. What does this ultrasound image suggest (200)?
ii. How should this condition be managed?

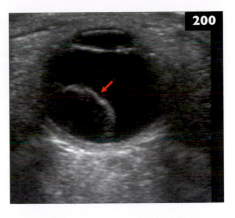

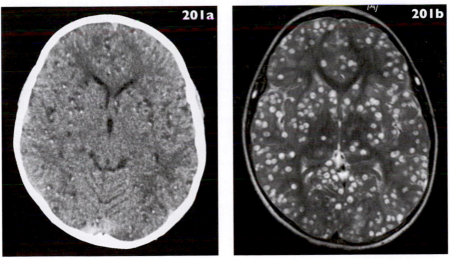

201 An 18-year-old male, who recently emigrated from Mexico, has had recent headaches and just awoke after a new-onset generalized, tonic–clonic seizure. He reported no previous medical problems and no illicit drug use. His neurologic examination was normal.
i. What diagnosis is suggested by these head CT and MR images (201a, b)?
ii. How should he be managed?

200 i. This is a large retinal detachment (RD) (arrow), which may begin in a small, localized area, but progressively enlarges, leading to vision loss and blindness. RD occurs with aging, trauma, myopia (present in two-thirds), after cataract surgery, and in proliferative retinopathy (e.g. diabetes mellitus, sickle cell disease). It is commonly preceded by a posterior vitreous detachment, with photopsia (flashes of light) and floaters appreciated. With RD, a dense peripheral visual shadow progressing centrally may be perceived, often described as curtain-like. Ultrasound and indirect ophthalmoscopy are valuable for diagnosis.

ii. RD is an ophthalmologic emergency. The goal is to find and seal all the RD areas, while releasing vitreous traction on the retina. Vitrectomy (removal of vitreous gel and replacement with gas or oil), cryotherapy (freezing), laser photocoagulation, scleral buckle surgery (banding the sclera to push the retinal wall inward, allowing reattachment), and pneumatic retinopexy (using injected gas to push the retina back down, followed by laser or cryotherapy) are techniques used for RD. Success is about 85% with one surgery, and may approach 100% with subsequent surgeries. Vision loss may be permanent if delay to repair is substantial.

201 i. Severe neurocysticercosis, the most common parasitic infection of the CNS worldwide and the main cause of acquired epilepsy in the developing world. It is seen everywhere due to ease of travel. Neurocysticercosis is caused by ingestion of eggs of the pig tapeworm (*Taenia solium*), usually from poorly cooked pork. Larvae develop, cross the intestinal wall, get into the bloodstream, and are transported to the CNS, muscle, and other tissues. Continued seeding from intestinal tapeworm infestation can be devastating. Many patients are asymptomatic, but headache, lightheadedness, and seizures are common. Altered mental status and hydrocephalus occur frequently, along with cerebrovascular accidents. Physical examination may show papilledema and almost any combination of neurologic findings. CT shows hypodense lesions with peripheral contrast enhancement as well as perilesional edema. Calcified parenchymal lesions are due to dead larvae. Hydrocephalus and diffuse cerebral edema may be present. Do CSF analysis if imaging studies are nondiagnostic, with special ELISAs having high sensitivity and specificity.

ii. Treatment depends on whether there are viable parasites. If not, anticonvulsant therapy is usually sufficient. For live parasites and ongoing brain inflammation, antiepileptics and a course of corticosteroids and/or immunosuppressants are recommended before anticysticercal therapy, which is usually with albendazole or praziquantel. Neurosurgical intervention may be necessary, with ventricular shunts and/or cyst resection for hydrocephalus due to intraventricular cysts.

202 A 37-year-old patient presented with a head injury after being an unrestrained front seat passenger in a motor vehicle collision. He arrived at the emergency department on a long backboard with cervical spine immobilization. He moaned when his sternum was rubbed and extended his arms and legs with this stimulation, while his eyes remained closed.
i. What is his Glascow Coma Score?
ii. What does this head CT image suggest (202)?

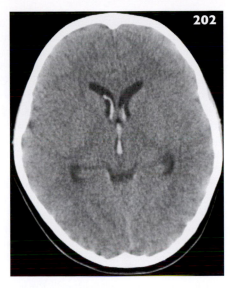

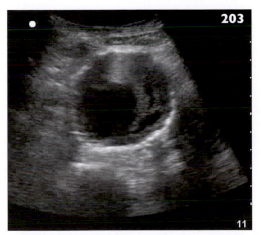

203 A 74-year-old male presented with severe back and abdominal pain. BP was 96/54 mmHg (12.8/7.2 kPa) with P 112 bpm. His abdomen was obese, but very tender around the umbilicus.
i. What does this ultrasound image suggest (203)?
ii. What management is indicated?

202 i. Many scoring systems attempt to quantify neurologic status following head trauma in ways that are simple, have high interobserver reproducibility, can be followed serially to recognize deterioration, and predict long-term outcome. The Glasgow Coma Score (GCS) scale has 3 components: eye response (1 = no eye opening; 2 = eyes opening to pain; 3 = eyes opening to speech; and 4 = eyes opening spontaneously); best verbal response (1 = no verbal response; 2 = incomprehensible sounds; 3 = inappropriate words; 4 = confused; 5 = oriented); and best motor response (1 = no motor response; 2 = decerebrate response or extension to pain; 3 = decorticate response or flexion to pain; 4 = withdraws to pain; 5 = localizes to pain; 6 = obeys commands). The scale has been adapted for pediatrics and included or modified into other scoring systems. Generally, brain injury is classified as severe (GCS ≤8), moderate (GCS 9–12), or minor (GCS ≥13), with related prognostic implications. The motor score appears to be the most important component. Unfortunately, many conditions interfere with the scale's ability to reflect accurately the severity of traumatic brain injury (e.g. alcohol and other drug intoxication, various metabolic disturbances). In addition, eye and spinal cord injury can make the score invalid. This patient has a GCS of 5.

ii. The CT image shows subtle traumatic subarachnoid hemorrhage with more visible intraventricular blood. Presently, supportive care is the only therapy available, although neurosurgical evaluation is imperative. Intracranial pressure monitoring is sometimes employed.

203 i. The ultrasound reveals a large abdominal aortic aneurysm (AAA), measuring approximately 7 cm in diameter. AAA is defined as a focal dilatation of at least 50% over normal aortic width, therefore usually 3 cm in diameter or more. This is the result of a degenerative process, usually attributed to atherosclerosis. Most AAAs are fusiform and infrarenal. Frequency rates increase with age (as high as 8% in elderly males). Incidental discovery with various imaging modalities is common. They are most commonly asymptomatic until leakage, when they may present with severe back and/or abdominal pain, often with a pulsatile abdominal mass.

ii. Hypotension and tachycardia with this ultrasound showing AAA should prompt immediate surgical consultation, along with appropriate monitoring and volume resuscitation. Blood samples for at least a CBC, along with type and crossmatch for multiple units of blood, should be sent to the laboratory. Further imaging with CT or MR is not necessary in this unstable patient, but might be helpful if hemodynamically stable. Do not let advanced imaging delay appropriate emergency care!

204 A 18-year-old female was in a motor vehicle collision and presented with severe left arm pain.
i. What common injuries are associated with this fracture (**204**)?
ii. How should this fracture be managed?

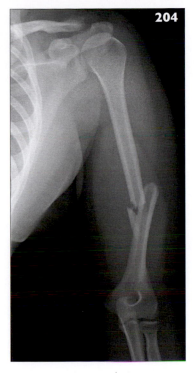

205 A 57-year-old female presented after leaving a theatre with severe pain in her right eye, visual blurring, and nausea. There was no history of trauma or previous eye complaints. She had a mid-position pupil, corneal clouding, and conjunctival injection.
i. What does this clinical scenario suggest?
ii. What diagnostic test is indicated?
iii. How should this patient be treated?

204 i. This is a midshaft humerus fracture, a frequent injury associated with motor vehicle collision, fall on an outstretched arm, and sport-related trauma. The most common complication is radial nerve injury, which is often reversible. The radial nerve innervates the dorsal extensor muscles of the wrist and fingers, so related loss of extension may occur with injury. Humerus fractures present with local ecchymoses, swelling, and pain with any movement. Simple radiographs are adequate for evaluation.

ii. About 80% of diaphyseal humerus fractures are nondisplaced. A coaptation splint is often reasonable management, where splint material is wrapped from the lateral shoulder, around the elbow, to the medial proximal humerus. Up to 30–40° of angulation is acceptable, as the shoulder has great ability to compensate. When the fracture cannot be stabilized adequately with splinting, surgical management may be required. An operation may also be necessary for open fractures, those with neurovascular injuries, or with associated large soft tissue defects. A floating elbow (ipsilateral humerus and forearm fractures) also requires operative repair. Intramedullary rods have become an effective tool for orthopedic stabilization of an increasing number of diaphyseal humerus fractures.

205 i. An acute attack of angle-closure glaucoma. This ocular emergency must be diagnosed and treated immediately to avoid permanent visual loss. Several anatomic abnormalities lead to anterior chamber crowding, predisposing to this problem. Attacks of angle-closure glaucoma commonly occur when susceptible patients enter a dark environment and dilate their pupils.

ii. Measurement of intraocular pressure (IOP). Tonometry using compressive (e.g. Schiotz) or applanation techniques are effective, with pressures >21 mmHg (2.8 kPa) abnormal. Symptomatic attacks of acute angle-closure glaucoma are usually associated with much higher pressures, which lead to retinal ischemia.

iii. Treatment includes rapid IOP reduction, suppression of inflammation, and reversal of angle closure. Topical beta blockers (e.g. timolol) enhance angle opening, as do alpha agonists (e.g. apraclonidine) drops. Topical steroids decrease inflammation and reduce optic nerve damage. Approximately 1 hour after beginning treatment, a miotic (e.g. pilocarpine), not useful initially due to pressure-related ischemic iris paralysis, will be of benefit. Hyperosmotic agents (e.g. mannitol) reduce IOP, while improving retinal perfusion. Acetazolamide orally or IV decreases aqueous humor production. Do not forget antiemetics and pain medications. Laser peripheral iridotomy is the most frequent definitive therapy of acute angle-closure glaucoma, usually done 24–48 hours after IOP is controlled. Involving the ophthalmologist early is important, particularly when serial IOP measurements do not rapidly improve. Argon laser peripheral iridoplasty and immediate paracentesis are alternative therapies in acute attacks.

206 A 39-year-old male was hurt in a motor vehicle collision and presented with acute right arm pain exacerbated by any movement.
i. What does this radiograph suggest (206a)?
ii. What is this injury associated with, and how is it treated?

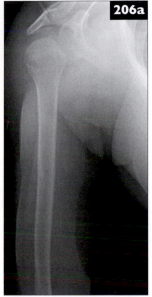

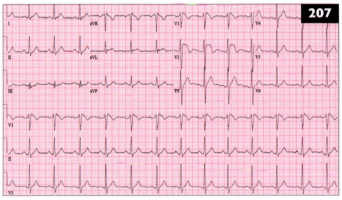

207 A 33-year-old male collapsed during a period of emotional upset and was found to be in ventricular fibrillation. Luckily, the emergency medical services response was very fast and the patient presented after a successful single attempt at defibrillation with normal neurologic function.
i. What does the ECG suggest happened (207)?
ii. How should he be managed?

206 i. This problem is easily missed, especially with altered mental status. There is an abnormally wide glenohumeral space. This finding might be dismissed as a positioning artifact. However, there is a posterior shoulder dislocation, which is rare (<5%). Anterior–posterior radiographs show a widened gleno-humeral joint and a symmetrically rounded humeral head, often termed the light bulb sign. A space between the anterior rim of the glenoid and the humeral head >6 mm is highly

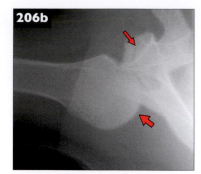

suggestive of posterior dislocation, as is a vacant anterior half of the glenoid fossa (**206b**, thin arrow). An axillary view shows the humeral head (**206b**, thick arrow) posterior to the empty glenoid fossa and overlying the acromion process. Posterior shoulder dislocations have an internally rotated arm fixed against the body, with pain on any motion.

ii. Axial loading of the adducted, internally rotated arm. Seizures and electrocution may also cause posterior shoulder dislocation, which can be bilateral. Closed reduction with adequate sedation is usually successful. Because diagnosis is frequently delayed for prolonged periods, and also for failed closed reduction, various surgical options may be necessary.

207 i. This is Brugada syndrome, a genetic disease inherited in an autosomal dominant manner. It is characterized by specific ECG abnormalities and increased risk of sudden death. Over 100 different mutations in seven genes have been reported in Brugada syndrome, most commonly to an alpha subunit of the sodium channel. It is more common in males, particularly Asians. Brugada syndrome has three distinct ECG types, with changes most visible in leads V_1–V_3. All types have coved-type or saddleback ST–T configurations, with J-point elevation of 2 mm or more and T waves that vary from negative to biphasic to positive. Brugada syndrome predisposes to polymorphic ventricular tachycardia and fibrillation. Responsible for about 4% of sudden nontraumatic deaths, it occurs at a mean age of about 40 years. Many clinical situations unmask or exacerbate ECG changes of Brugada syndrome, including hypokalemia or hyperkalemia, hypercalcemia, alcohol consumption, and use of certain drugs (e.g. cocaine) or medications (e.g. procainamide). Occasionally, drug challenge will unmask the ECG pattern, and cardiologists may also use electro-physiological studies to determine arrhythmia inducibility.

ii. No pharmacologic therapy has been shown to reduce incidence of ventricular tachycardia or fibrillation in Brugada syndrome. Only implantation of a cardiac defibrillator reduces mortality.

208 A 24-year-old female presented with severe right thigh pain and was thought to have cellulitis.
i. Should further evaluation be done?
ii. What evidence-based therapy is indicated?

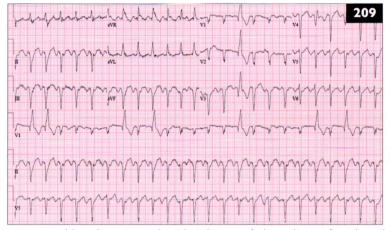

209 A 55-year-old male presented with 2 hours of chest discomfort described as tightness, along with severe shortness of breath. He had a history of hypertension, heart failure, COPD, and medication noncompliance. BP was 124/80 mmHg (16.5/10.7 kPa) with P 148 bpm.
i. What does this ECG suggest (**209**)?
ii. Should this be treated as a STEMI?

208 i. Distinguishing cellulitis from a significant underlying skin abscess is often difficult using clinical features alone. In immunosuppressed patients, due to disease or medications, inflammatory response may be minimal. Needle aspiration is a diagnostic technique that may be helpful if purulent fluid is obtained, but the false-negative rate is significant. Ultrasound using a high-frequency probe can help recognize collections of purulent fluid (208,

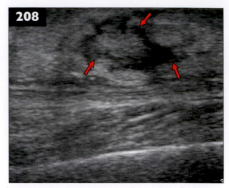

arrows) in the subcutaneous tissue. *Staphylococcus aureus* causes the overwhelming majority of these skin abscesses, with an increasing number of these organisms methicillin resistant.

ii. 'To cut is to cure' is a relevant adage in the immunocompetent patient with simple skin abscesses. Thorough incision with drainage is all that is usually necessary, even with large abscesses. Although abscess cavity packing is common, there is no evidence to support this practice. Primary incision closure in abscess management is also controversial. Abscess cultures and/or antibiotic coverage are generally not necessary unless the patient is immunocompromised or has other systemic indications (e.g. sepsis). Do not forget to explore for and remove foreign bodies. Appropriate pain medications must not be forgotten.

209 i. This is a rapid, regular, narrow-complex tachycardia at about 150 bpm with some intermittent fusion beats. Whenever we see a narrow-complex tachycardia at about 150 bpm, atrial flutter with 2:1 atrioventricular block should be strongly considered. It is very difficult to confirm flutter waves on this ECG. Vagal maneuvers or adenosine injection may be used to increase the degree of atrioventricular block and to help clarify flutter waves.

ii. It certainly looks as though 3 mm or so of ST segment elevation is present in leads II, III, and aVF, which in this situation would trigger treatment as a STEMI. However, these are actually flutter waves superimposed on normal ST segments. Calcium channel blockers, digoxin, amiodarone, or magnesium are among agents generally helpful for rate control in atrial flutter. Although beta blockers are also very effective for rate control, other agents are likely better tolerated in this clinical setting given the history of heart failure and COPD.

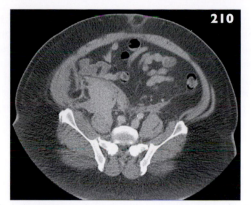

210 A 56-year-old male presented with right groin and lower abdominal pain that had increased since a cardiac catheterization done 5 days previously. His vital signs were normal. His right lower abdomen was mildly tender and he had minimal ecchymoses over the right proximal thigh at the puncture site. There was no local bruit or evidence of limb ischemia.
i. What does this CT image suggest may be going on here (210)?
ii. How should he be managed?

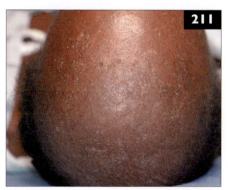

211 A 78-year-old male had chronic hypertension and diabetes mellitus, but had not seen a physician for years. He presented with weakness and shortness of breath. BP was 196/110 mmHg (26.1/14.7 kPa) with P 64 bpm, RR 28/min.
i. What does this photograph show (211)?
ii. What emergency evaluation and management is indicated?

210 i. The CT image demonstrates a large right retroperitoneal hemorrhage, consistent with ongoing arterial leakage. The most common complication of femoral artery cannulation for cardiac catheterization is simple subcutaneous hematoma, occurring in up to 10%. More serious but infrequent complications include arteriovenous fistula, pseudoaneurysm, retroperitoneal hemorrhage, limb ischemia, ongoing external bleeding, and local infection. Among iatrogenic femoral or external iliac artery injuries, pseudoaneurysm is most frequent, with incidence up to 0.5% after diagnostic angiography (higher with stent placement). Pseudo-aneurysm (false aneurysm) is a hematoma resulting from continued arterial leak. This forms outside the arterial wall, and may continue to expand over time. Here, history and physical examination tend to exclude the other listed entities. Ultrasound is an effective diagnostic modality. CT is useful in many cases.
ii. Volume resuscitation and blood transfusion are initiated as necessary. Small pseudoaneurysms generally close without therapy. Local compression, manually or by various commercial devices, resolves many others. Ultrasound-guided compression, often with percutaneous thrombin injection, is frequently employed. Angiography through the contralateral femoral artery allows crossover access, with contrast used to define site of bleeding or stenosis. Balloon tamponade over the bleeding site, intravascular thrombin, and stent deployment are some of the techniques used to manage these complications. Open surgical repair remains a definitive option if the above techniques fail.

211 i. Uremic frost, a rare dermatologic manifestation of severe azotemia, with powdery deposits of urea and uric acid salts on the skin. Uremic frost is rarely seen today because of early dialysis in renal insufficiency.
ii. Rapid evaluation for hyperkalemia, as well as heart failure due to fluid overload, is important. ECG and chest radiographs, as well as rapid measurement of serum potassium and renal indices, are necessary. These problems should be managed and the patient evaluated for dialysis indications.

212 A 27-year-old female presented with a severe bifrontal headache and nasal congestion, which began as a minor upper respiratory infection and had become progressively worse despite a week of antibiotics. She had some mild, nontender, bilateral periorbital edema.

i. What does this radiograph suggest (**212**)?

ii. How should she be managed?

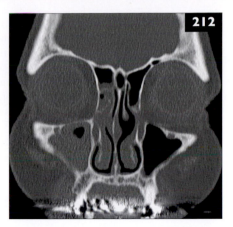

213 A 28-year-old male was found unconscious at home. He had a history of AIDS and was on multiple unknown medications. No further history was available. BP was 150/90 mmHg (20.0/12.0 kPa), P 112 bpm, RR 36/min, and T 37.9°C. His P_{ox} would not register. His bedside glucose was 7.3 mmol/l (132 mg/dl). Lungs were clear, and cardiac examination showed a regular S1 and S2 with II/VI systolic murmur. He was nonverbal, but had localized pain with sternal rub and moved all his extremities. Arterial blood gas analysis showed a pH of 7.08, arterial carbon dioxide of 12 mmHg (1.6 kPa), and arterial oxygen of 97 mmHg (12.9 kPa).

i. Is there anything else that should be noted about this blood, and why won't his P_{ox} register (**213**)?

ii. How should he be treated?

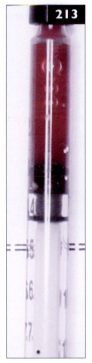

212 i. This patient has evidence of rhinosinusitis, with mucoperiosteal thickening and fluid in the right maxillary and ethmoid sinuses. Acute rhinosinusitis is most commonly precipitated by a viral upper respiratory infection or by allergic rhinitis. Typically, the patient presents with nasal congestion, purulent nasal discharge, cough, headache, and facial pain. Diagnosis is clinical, with imaging rarely necessary unless there is suspicion of orbital, intracranial, or bony extension. Failure to respond to conservative therapy might be an additional imaging indication.

ii. Most acute rhinosinusitis is viral. Symptomatic management using nasal corticosteroids is the most efficient approach to uncomplicated rhinosinusitis. Antibiotics should be reserved for those with severe or rapidly worsening symptoms as well as those who have complications, are immunocompromised, or fail to respond to conservative therapy. Rarely, otolaryngology specialty assistance may be needed for sinus drainage (often endoscopically) or other problems in complex cases.

213 i. The blood looks like some red, flavored water. His arterial blood gas revealed a hemoglobin level of 14 g/l (1.4 g/dl). (Initially, the hospital laboratory refused to release the result, stating it was 'incompatible with life'. They were mostly correct.) P_{ox} is based on two physical principles, pulsatile blood flow and the different absorption spectra of oxyhemoglobin and deoxygenated hemoglobin. Studies have found that P_{ox} readings are highly inaccurate and may be unobtainable with hemoglobin below about 30 g/l (3 g/dl).

ii. This patient needs some blood now! Each unit of packed RBCs will raise his hemoglobin by about 10 g/l (1 g/dl) and he needs fairly rapid infusion of 4–6 units. A search for a source of acute blood loss is important. However, it was determined in this case, after bone marrow biopsy and medication discontinuation, that severe marrow suppression due to HIV medications was the cause. (He had a macrocytic anemia.)

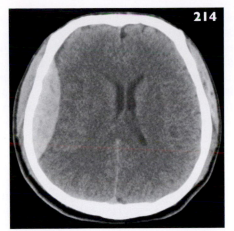

214 A 25-year-old male was struck in the head with a heavy object 1 hour ago. He presented confused and agitated. Examination revealed a dilated, sluggish right pupil and decreased movement on his left side.
i. What is the diagnosis based on this CT image (214)?
ii. How should this problem be managed?

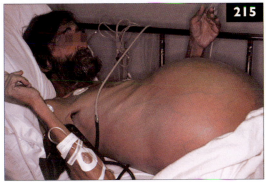

215 A 63-year-old male presented with progressive abdominal swelling (215), which was associated with loss of appetite and difficulty breathing.
i. What are common causes of this clinical finding?
ii. How should the patient be managed?

214 i. A large epidural hematoma (blood between inner skull and dural membrane) caused by direct focal trauma. Loss of consciousness with return to normal alertness and then deterioration, the so-called 'lucid interval', occurs in about 15%. Headache, seizure, vomiting, and alterations of consciousness are the main symptoms. Underlying brain is often minimally injured. Examination reveals local scalp contusion or laceration, frequently with bony step-off. A dilated or sluggish pupil ipsilateral to the injury can be present, as may contralateral hemiplegia. With progression, due to increased intracranial pressure and transtentorial brain herniation, both pupils become dilated and fixed, with deterioration of consciousness and posturing. An immediate noncontrast brain CT scan is the diagnostic modality of choice. Epidural hematoma appears biconcave and rarely crosses suture lines because of tight dural attachments.

ii. For symptomatic epidural hematoma, rapid sequence intubation with paralysis and ventilation to a CO_2 of 30–35 mmHg (4.0–4.7 kPa) is indicated. The head of the bed should be elevated 30–45° and seizure prophylaxis (e.g. phenytoin) given. Consider mannitol, which reduces intracranial pressure by osmotically decreasing cerebral edema while increasing brain perfusion. Rapid decompression leads to an excellent prognosis if accomplished before neurologic deterioration. It is indicated in hematomas larger than 30 cm^3 or if the patient has a Glascow Coma Score <9 with anisocoria. Epidural hematomas <30 cm^3 with <15 mm thickness and <5 mm midline shift may be selectively managed nonoperatively with serial neuroimaging and close observation in a neurosurgical center. Emergency trepination is rarely necessary.

215 i. Abdominal distension has many causes, but in this malnourished male with subtle gynecomastia, prominent superficial veins, and tense abdominal swelling, it is due to a tremendous amount of ascites (accumulation of fluid in the peritoneal cavity, most often due to severe liver disease [e.g. cirrhosis]). It may vary from unappreciable to massive. Physical examination findings in ascites include shifting dullness (changing percussion note in the flanks with position changes), fluid wave, and distension. Ultrasound is very effective at confirming ascites. Diagnostic paracentesis should usually be done for new ascites, with cell counts, albumin level, and Gram stain with culture. If the serum/ascites albumin ratio is <1, the fluid is exudative, making malignancy or infection more likely.

ii. Therapeutic paracentesis gives prompt symptomatic relief of tense ascites and may help with diagnosis. Further treatment is etiology dependent. Dietary salt restriction, antialdosterone diuretics (e.g. spironolactone), and, occasionally, shunt procedures (e.g. transjugular intrahepatic portosystemic shunt) are used for ascites.

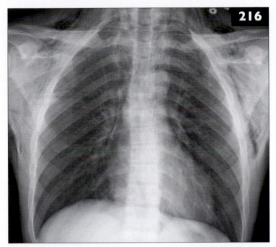

216 A 32-year-old male was involved in a motor vehicle collision and had multiple injuries. He had diffuse chest pain with shortness of breath. There was no chest wound.
i. What does this chest radiograph suggest (**216**)?
ii. How should he be managed?

217 A 43-year-old female presented with severe dyspnea along with cyanosis of her tongue, fingers, and toes. She reported a previous history of bacterial endocarditis and had mechanical tricuspid valve replacement several years ago. She had failed to take her anticoagulant medication for several months. Her oxygen saturation was 70% and improved little with 100% oxygen via face mask. She had no heart murmur. Her chest radiograph demonstrated a metallic tricuspid valve, without evidence of cardiomegaly or pulmonary edema.
i. What do you think is going on?
ii. How should this patient be diagnosed and treated?

216 i. There is diffuse, uncontained air in abnormal places, including the neck, supraclavicular fossae, and chest subcutaneous tissue as well as outlining the trachea, right mainstem bronchus, and pectoral muscles. This is traumatic pneumo-mediastinum, or mediastinal emphysema, with air leak usually from alveolar, airway, or esophageal rupture. Most cases are due to sudden increased pressure within the lungs or airways. Other etiologies include positive pressure ventilation, Valsalva mechanism (e.g. excessive coughing, sneezing, or vomiting), rapid altitude ascent (e.g. SCUBA diving), recreational drug use (e.g. crack cocaine), abdominal visceral perforation, pneumothorax, external wounds, and some rare diseases. Pneumomediastinum may be asymptomatic, but pleuritic chest pain, dyspnea, subcutaneous emphysema, and throat pain are common. A crunching sound auscultated over the heart synchronous with the heartbeat, called Hamman's crunch, may be appreciated.

ii. Search for a cause is dictated by the mechanism of injury and clinical presentation. CT, direct bronchoscopy, esophagoscopy, and/or contrast swallow is often necessary. Pneumomediastinum usually has a self-limiting course and is typically managed with analgesia and observation. Deterioration should prompt a search for missed etiologies. Surgical intervention or catheter drainage is rarely necessary, usually only in hemodynamically compromised patients. Pneumomediastinum may take 10 or more days to resolve.

217 i. This is an interesting case. The fact that her oxygen saturation does not improve with high-flow oxygen therapy is very suggestive of right-to-left shunting. Considerations were a thrombosed tricuspid valve with shunt through a patent foramen ovale, or possibly a large pulmonary embolism with similar shunting.

ii. The diagnosis was confirmed by transthoracic echocardiography, which showed a thrombosed mechanical tricuspid valve, with presumed patent foramen ovale. Thrombolysis was indicated and successful here. Surgical valve repair or replacement would have been necessary if thrombolysis was unsuccessful. Percutaneous device closure of her patent foramen ovale was done because of concern about future paradoxical arterial embolization.

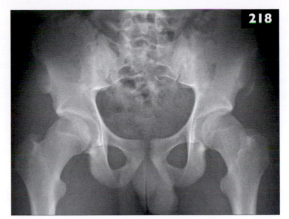

218 An 18-year-old male presented with sudden left hip pain after beginning a sprint.
i. What does this radiograph display (218)?
ii. How should he be treated?

219 A 25-year-old woman was involved in a high-speed motor vehicle collision. She was approximately 34 weeks pregnant. She had a minor head contusion without other visible injuries, but she also had moderate abdominal pain and tenderness. BP was 96/62 mmHg (12.8/8.3 kPa) with P 112 bpm.
i. What are the priorities in this patient?
ii. What is the best evaluation for placental abruption?

218 i. An apophyseal injury, an avulsion of bone or cartilage where tendon attaches. These occur in skeletally immature athletes, usually between 13 and 23 years old, most frequently caused by forceful associated muscle contraction. Pelvic apophyseal injuries occur at the anterior superior iliac spine (as in this case) where the sartorius muscle attaches, anterior inferior iliac spine, ischial tuberosity, iliac crest, and lesser trochanter. Apophysitis is a chronic inflammation due to repeated traction at tendon insertion sites in these patients. Perhaps the most famous apophysitis is Osgood–Schlatter disease at the tibial tuberosity of the knee where the patellar tendon inserts.

ii. Most of these injuries are treated conservatively, with rest and no weight bearing. Occasionally, orthopedic surgery is needed, so referral is appropriate.

219 i. ABC, with appropriate monitoring of mother and child, are the main priorities. Best management for the fetus is optimal maternal resuscitation. Intravascular volume is increased up to 50% during pregnancy, so hemorrhagic volume depletion may be very significant despite fairly normal maternal vital signs. FAST ultrasound evaluation should be done promptly to search for intra-abdominal hemorrhage. Evaluation of the fetus is an added benefit. Main considerations in blunt trauma during pregnancy include placental abruption, amniotic fluid embolism, uterine injury, premature rupture of membranes, and isoimmunization.

ii. Traumatic placental abruption is most commonly due to motor vehicle collision, fall, or domestic violence; it may occur with minor trauma. Electronic fetal monitoring remains the most accurate method to recognize fetal distress after trauma. CT is sensitive for placental abruption, while ultrasound may miss it, particularly when small. CBC, coagulation studies, blood type and screen (do not forget an anti-rhesus D-protein immunoglobulin injection if rhesus-negative mother), and Kleihauer–Betke testing (looks for fetal cells in adult circulation) are appropriate.

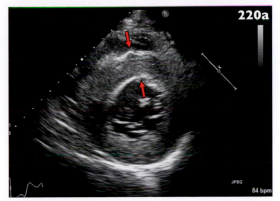

220 A 41-year-old male presented with increasing dyspnea on exertion along with sudden onset of intermittent palpitations. He had no chest pain. Echocardiography was carried out.
i. What does this short-axis cardiac view echocardiographic image suggest (220a)?
ii. How should he be managed?

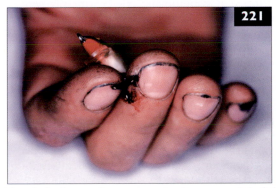

221 A 27-year-old male had an unfortunate misadventure while fishing (221). How would you manage this problem?

220 i. The thickened inter-ventricular septum (220a, arrows) compared with the posterior myocardial wall suggests hypertrophic cardio-myopathy (HCM). Inherited in an autosomal-dominant manner, this disease is attributed to one of several genetic mutations encoding for sarcomere pro-

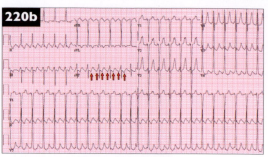

teins. Myocardial cell alignment is in disarray, which affects heart mechanical and electrical functions. HCM is a significant cause of sudden cardiac death, particularly in young athletes. About 25% of HCM patients have left ventricle outflow obstruction at rest. Others develop dynamic outflow obstruction with exertion, usually due to systolic anterior motion of the anterior leaflet of the mitral valve, which impedes cardiac output. Many patients are asymptomatic. Symptoms correlate poorly with amount of outflow obstruction and include dyspnea, chest pain, palpitations, lightheadedness, and/or syncope as well as sudden cardiac death. Their systolic murmur is exacerbated with increased outflow obstruction, achieved by maneuvers that decrease preload, increase contractility, or decrease afterload. Echocardiography, cardiac MRI, and catheterization are diagnostic. Genetic testing is important for family members and in equivocal cases.

ii. Treatment is directed at symptomatic relief, primarily with beta blockers (e.g. atenolol) or calcium channel blockers (e.g. verapamil). Atrial flutter (220b, arrows) or fibrillation is a common cause of deterioration in HCM, as in this case. Risk assessment for sudden cardiac death is important, with defibrillator placement often life saving. Surgical septal myectomy is useful in patients who remain symptomatic despite medical therapy, and alcohol ablation of the septum may also be effective in selected cases.

221 Fishhook injuries are fairly common worldwide. While impalement by all three barbs of this treble hook provides a bit more of a challenge, where the hook is embedded determines the complexity of removal. For example, a fishhook in the eyeball requires ophthalmologic consultation. In general, fishhooks are most easily removed by rotating the barb forward through the skin, cutting it off with wire cutters, and rotating the barbless hook back out. Here, after a digital block to the involved fingers, the three shanks of the treble hook were separately cut at the base, with each removed by advancing the hooks out. Other techniques for fishhook removal have been described.

222 A 50-year-old intoxicated female fell about 4–6 meters (15–20 feet) off a balcony when she tried to reach for a pack of cigarettes that fell out of her shirt pocket. There was initial loss of consciousness, but she presented neurologically intact with a complaint of severe left-sided chest pain.

i. What does this chest radiograph demonstrate (222a)?

ii. How should this patient be managed?

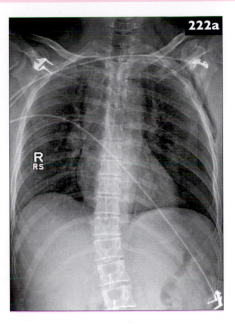

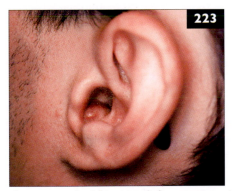

223 A 19-year-old male presented with severe left ear pain, without any history of trauma.

i. What is this condition (223)?

ii. How is it treated?

222 i. Multiple left rib fractures, subcutaneous emphysema in the left upper chest and neck (thin arrows), along with a small left pneumothorax (thick arrows). Evidence of pneumomediastinum (arrowheads) along the descending aorta and thoracolumbar scoliosis is also present. CT confirmed these findings with more detail (222b).

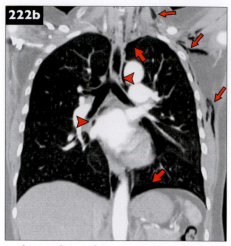

ii. This patient needs a full trauma evaluation along with appropriate stabilization. Pneumothorax (air in the pleural space) may be closed (simple), communicate through a wound to the atmosphere (open), or be associated with mediastinal shift (tension). Small simple pneumothoraces may gradually resolve without therapy. Larger pneumothoraces need drainage, especially those with associated respiratory distress or requiring positive pressure ventilation and/or general anesthesia. Open and tension pneumothoraces, as well as those with associated hemothorax, also need evacuation. Emergency venting of tension pneumothorax is indicated with clinical suspicion and evidence of hypoperfusion, usually with a long needle or catheter introduced above the third rib anteriorly in the mid-clavicular line. Various thoracostomy tubes and catheters are used for pneumothorax, with attachment to water-sealed suction devices. Larger tubes are used with suspected hemopneumothorax. Remember to cover the wound in open pneumothorax. Pneumomediastinum in general requires no treatment.

223 i. An otofuruncle, a painful localized infection of an external ear canal hair follicle. It is generally caused by *Staphylococcus aureus*, but occasionally due to *Pseudomonas aeruginosa*. Infection in the external ear canal can quickly spread, particularly in diabetics and other immunocompromised patients. Pain, itching, and decreased hearing are the main symptoms of external ear boils.

ii. Most otofuruncles are self-limiting and resolve on their own. Pain medication and warm compresses to the external ear may help. Antibiotics may be necessary for spreading infections or in immunocompromised patients. Incision and drainage is occasionally necessary.

224 A 70-year-old female presented with acute onset of severe pain in both lower extremities. She had a history of recently diagnosed lung cancer and was preparing for chemotherapy. She had been having an increase of her chronic headaches, but her brain MRI was normal. Hemoglobin was 80 g/l (8.0 g/dl). Her legs and feet were pale and cold, with absent posterior tibial and dorsalis pedis arterial pulses bilaterally (**224**).

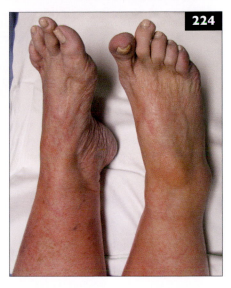

i. Considering the patient has started a new headache medicine (she does not recall the name), can you figure out what is happening here?

ii. How should she be treated?

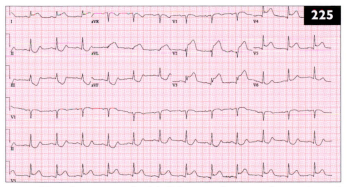

225 A 68-year-old male presented with 2 hours of severe chest pain and shortness of breath. He had no known heart disease, but he had longstanding hypertension, diabetes mellitus, and hyperlipidemia. BP was 76/56 mmHg (10.1/7.5 kPa), P 124 bpm, and RR 36/min. Lung examination revealed diffuse inspiratory crackles and cardiac examination included an S_3 gallop with jugular venous distension, but no pedal edema.

i. What does this ECG suggest is the problem (**225**)?

ii. What management is indicated?

224 i. This is a fascinating case. The patient has acute bilateral peripheral arterial insufficiency, with skin pallor, toe cyanosis, and severe pain. It is a bit unusual to see acute, isolated bilateral lower extremity hypoperfusion, and one tends to think about some event above the aortic bifurcation. However, in this case the patient had begun taking an ergotamine and caffeine combination medication and apparently she was dosing it more frequently than recommended. This led to ergotamine-induced vasoconstriction.

ii. With a vasodilating agent and some crystalloid volume infusion to maintain perfusion. Nitrates, calcium channel blockers, and angiotensin-converting enzyme inhibitors are some of the medications that may help improve acute symptoms. She may require peripheral arterial studies, usually Doppler ultrasound, if there is not prompt relief with these medications. Her anemia probably contributes to the problem and should be addressed. Do not forget, she needs a new headache medication!

225 i. The ECG demonstrates an acute anterolateral myocardial infarction. In the setting of hypoperfusion with clinical evidence of acute pulmonary edema, this is cardiogenic shock. Diagnostic criteria for cardiogenic shock include sustained hypotension (systolic BP <90 mmHg [12.0 kPa]) lasting more than 30 minutes with evidence of tissue hypoperfusion, along with either pulmonary edema or high left ventricular (LV) filling pressure. The most common cause of cardiogenic shock is acute myocardial infarction. It also occurs due to acute valvular failure (e.g. papillary muscle dysfunction leading to acute mitral regurgitation), as well as with ventricular septal or free wall rupture due to infarction. Certain medications lead to cardiogenic shock, particularly overdose with calcium channel blockers or beta blockers. Systemic infection, pulmonary embolism, endocarditis, and viral myocarditis are other culprits. Right ventricular infarct and cardiac tamponade, which cause hypotension through decreased LV filling volumes, may be confused with cardiogenic shock.

ii. Start treatment by establishing adequate oxygenation. Repeated crystalloid boluses of 250 ml or more improve perfusion in about 25% of patients with suspected cardiogenic shock due to acute myocardial infarction. Vasopressors (e.g. norepinephrine) may be necessary to improve BP, but all increase myocardial work. Percutaneous interventions or emergency bypass grafting are treatments of choice to re-establish coronary perfusion. Thrombolytics have less utility in cardiogenic shock. Intra-aortic balloon pump use may improve perfusion in this setting.

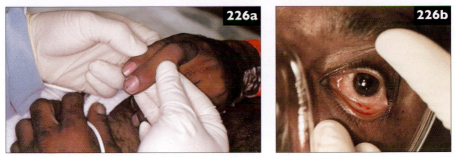

226 A 39-year-old male arrived unconscious after supposedly overdosing on IV narcotics. However, he did not respond to aggressive naloxone dosing and he had these clinical findings (226a, b).
i. What do you think is going on?
ii. What confirmatory tests and treatments are indicated?

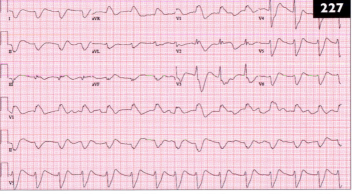

227 A 59-year-old female with a history of diabetes mellitus and hypertension presented with weakness, hypotension, and shortness of breath.
i. What does this ECG suggest (227)?
ii. How should this condition be managed?

226 i. This patient has subconjunctival petechiae and fingernail splinter hemorrhages, making endocarditis likely in this IV drug user. One must consider other etiologies for his altered mental status (e.g. hypoglycemia, head trauma), but an intracranial catastrophe (e.g. meningitis or ruptured mycotic aneurysm secondary to endocarditis) is a distinct possibility.

ii. Attention to airway management and primary resuscitation is the first priority. Because endocarditis seems highly probable, early antibiotics to cover likely pathogens are important. *Staphylococcus aureus* and *S. epidermidis* are the most common organisms in IV drug abusers, with infective endocarditis most frequently involving the tricuspid valve in this group. Gram-negative and anaerobic organisms should also be initially covered after collection of several blood cultures to help identify the causative organisms. Heart murmurs are infrequently heard in right-sided endocarditis due to low right-sided pressure gradients. CT neuroimaging, followed by lumbar puncture as indicated (if there is no evidence of brain mass effect), should be carried out promptly. Echocardiography should be performed to look for heart valve vegetations, myocardial abscesses, and other cardiac pathology.

227 i. Severe hyperkalemia, a life-threatening condition that can quickly deteriorate to ventricular fibrillation or asystole. Tissue breakdown (e.g. sepsis, rhabdomyolysis), certain medications (e.g. potassium supplements, angiotensin-converting enzyme inhibitors), and hormonal deficiencies (e.g. adrenal insufficiency) are common causes. Significant renal insufficiency is usually present. Symptomatic hyperkalemia often presents with muscle weakness, fatigue, nausea, heart failure, and various cardiac arrhythmias. For prompt diagnosis, consider hyperkalemia early in hypoperfusion states, muscle weakness, or various cardiac arrhythmias. Rapid laboratory testing is critical (usually symptomatic with K >6.5 mmol/l [mEq/l]). The ECG is a quick screening tool, with tall, narrow-based precordial T waves highly suggestive. PR prolongation with P wave disappearance and QRS complex widening are also frequent. This patient shows irregular, wide QRS and T waves, the so-called 'sine wave' changes ominous for severe hyperkalemia with impending cardiac arrest. (Serum K was 8.2 mmol/l [mEq /l]). Rarely, the ECG may be normal even in severe hyperkalemia.

ii. Treat immediately if reasonable clinical suspicion in a symptomatic patient or for serum K >6.5 mmol/l (mEq/l), particularly if hypoperfusion or cardiac arrhythmias exists. IV calcium chloride or calcium gluconate antagonizes potassium effects on the heart rapidly. IV sodium bicarbonate and/or dextrose with insulin help by shifting potassium into cells, as do nebulized beta-sympathomimetic agents (and IV epinephrine). Intubation with hyperventilation also shifts potassium intracellularly. Increase potassium excretion with loop diuretics (e.g. furosemide). Ion-binding agents (e.g. sodium polystyrene sulfonate) have minimal utility. Dialysis remains the long-term solution in renal insufficiency.

228 A 48-year-old male was assaulted and pushed to the ground 4 hours ago. He struck his head and hurt his neck. He initially could not move his right side. On presentation, he was intoxicated, which made examination difficult. He had a forehead hematoma. Strength testing was 3 of 5 in his right upper and 4 of 5 in his left upper extremity, with normal strength in both lower extremities.
i. What is the problem, and what is the likely etiology?
ii. What treatments are useful in this clinical situation?

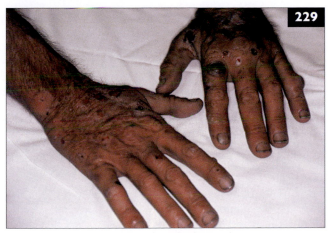

229 A 47-year-old alcoholic presented with this rash (229) in sun-exposed areas only, which had occurred in the past. He had chronic hepatitis C.
i. What is this rash?
ii. Are antibiotics indicated?

228 i. The clinical scenario suggests acute cervical injury with central cord syndrome (CCS), usually occurring in older patients with cervical spondolysis. CCS is characterized by greater upper than lower extremity weakness, often with bladder and/or anal sphincter dysfunction, along with variable sensory deficits. Most commonly caused by cervical hyperextension, CCS results from cord concussion or contusion rather than disruption. Prognosis is generally good. However, recent autopsy data suggest frequent bleeding into the central cord in some cases, with associated

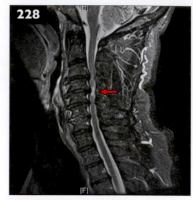

axonal disruption that may lead to permanent disability. The corticospinal tracts provide motor information to the body and are arranged from sacral on the periphery to cervical centrally. MRI most accurately evaluates suspected spinal cord injuries and here confirms severe stenosis from third to fifth cervical levels, with internal cord signal abnormality at the fourth cervical level (**228**, arrow).

ii. Treatment involves physical therapy to preserve range of motion and mobility. Surgery is rarely indicated, but may be considered when spinal cord compression or spine instability persists or if neurologic deficits progress. Several studies have suggested that IV methylprednisolone within the first few hours of injury may improve neurologic recovery in blunt spinal cord trauma, but design and statistical flaws make these findings controversial.

229 i. Porphyria cutanea tarda, a disease caused by low levels of one of the enzymes responsible for heme production, uroporphyrinogen decarboxalase. It is inherited in 20%, but sporadic in 80%. Porphyria cutanea tarda presents as a photodermatitis, with blisters, erosions, and hyperpigmentation on sun-exposed skin. It heals with scarring. It occurs in liver disease, particularly with hepatitis C, as well as in alcohol abuse, estrogen use, excess iron retention, or exposure to chlorinated cyclic hydrocarbons. Laboratory testing reveals high levels of uroporphyrinogen in the urine, although the rash itself is usually suggestive.

ii. This is not an infectious disease, so antibiotics are not indicated. Avoidance of inducers like alcohol, estrogen, iron, or chlorinated cyclic hydrocarbons, as well as limiting sunlight exposure, may help control the rash. Porphyria cutanea tarda is a chronic condition. Therapies to reduce excess iron and, occasionally, low-dose antimalarials have been used to control the rash.

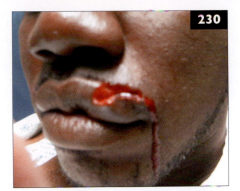

230 A 23-year-old male was allegedly assaulted and believed that a ring attached to the fist of his attacker lacerated his lip (**230**). He had no other injury. How should this laceration be managed?

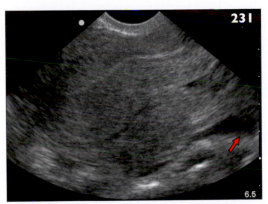

231 A 18-year-old female presented with acute lower abdominal pain and vaginal spotting. She was unsure about the time of her last menstrual period, but she denied any sexual activity. However, her quantitative beta-hCG level was 2,200 mIU/ml. BP was 88/60 mmHg (11.7/8.0 kPa) with P 128 bpm.
i. What does her ultrasound image suggest (**231**)?
ii. What management is indicated here?

230 Verify that the teeth and maxilla are not fractured and that no other associated injuries exist. This wound lends itself to anesthesia with an infraorbital nerve block, done either intraorally or extraorally. Slow injection of warm, buffered anesthetic reduces local anesthesia-related pain. Alignment of the vermillion border will optimize cosmetic repair, which may be facilitated by using an indelible marker to tag each side precisely prior to the procedure. Copious irrigation is important and clean water under pressure is as effective as saline. Use clean gloves; sterile gloves add little. Deep absorbable sutures take the tension off surface ones and improve final results. Absorbable surface stitches can be used, but these may dissolve more rapidly than desired in this potentially high wound tension setting. An emollient ointment (with or without antibiotics) may improve cosmesis. Take pride in a careful, nontraumatic repair technique. Often, pre- and postprocedural photographs improve patient appreciation of your excellent repair. Since the lip is a muscle that generates considerable tension, early suture removal may lead to wound repair failure here, so waiting 6–7 days before removal is usually appropriate (sometimes longer in elderly patients and in those with health problems or medications that delay wound healing).

231 i. The ultrasound image shows an empty uterus, with fluid in the rectovaginal space (arrow). There are large variations in normal beta-hCG levels for any given time in pregnancy. Levels generally double every 2–3 days up to 8–10 weeks of pregnancy and then gradually decline. Transvaginal ultrasound can detect an intrauterine pregnancy as early as 38 days after the last menstrual period. With a quantitative beta-hCG above approximately 1,500 mIU/ml, a transvaginal ultrasound in skilled hands should reveal an intrauterine pregnancy. Similarly, a level >6,500 mIU/ml should show this on transabdominal ultrasound. These respective quantitative beta-hCG levels are called discriminatory levels. In the setting of an empty uterus on transvaginal ultrasound with quantitative beta-hCG above the discriminatory level, ectopic pregnancy is likely. Associated free fluid in the rectovaginal space makes it even more probable. The classic triad of ectopic pregnancy is pain, amenorrhea, and vaginal bleeding, but less than half present in the typical manner.

ii. This patient has evidence of hemodynamic instability in the setting of a likely ectopic pregnancy. She needs immediate obstetric consultation. Volume resuscitation along with CBC, type and crossmatch, and appropriate hemodynamic monitoring should be carried out while awaiting definitive surgical therapy.

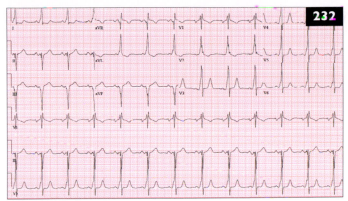

232 A 27-year-old male presented with recurrent, episodic heart racing, which he attributed to an unknown pill a friend had just given him. His heart rate was normal on arrival. An ECG was obtained (**232**).
i. Do you think the pill has anything to do with his problem?
ii. Does he require any therapy?

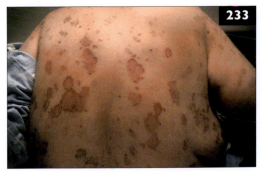

233 A 74-year-old female had a dry, itchy rash (**233**), which was getting worse despite frequent bathing.
i. What is this rash?
ii. How should it be treated?

232 i. The ECG demonstrates underlying Wolff–Parkinson–White (WPW) syndrome, a congenital problem where accessory pathways exist between atria and ventricles. Typical findings include slurred initial QRS complex upstroke (delta wave), along with shortened PR interval, prolongation of QRS complex, and aberrant ventricular repolarization. An accessory pathway may not always manifest itself on standard ECG, occasionally unmasked only in certain clinical situations. Most accessory pathways allow both antegrade and retrograde conduction. Certain medications may accelerate accessory pathway conduction, particularly calcium channel blockers, beta blockers, and digoxin. The unknown pill may have contributed to his new palpitations.

ii. Presently, the patient requires only observation. If a tachyarrhythmia develops, the main principle is to slow conduction down the accessory pathway more than down the atrioventricular node. Cardioversion/defibrillation equipment should be immediately available. Narrow-complex, regular tachycardia can usually be resolved by IV adenosine. Any irregular rhythm, whether the QRS complex is narrow or wide, suggests atrial flutter or fibrillation. Here, standard therapy with calcium channel blockers, beta blockers, or digoxin will block the atrioventricular node, but may increase accessory pathway conduction and ventricular rate, leading to deterioration and often to ventricular fibrillation. Thus, irregular tachyarrhythmias in WPW syndrome should be treated with electricity, although a trial of procainamide or amiodarone is reasonable if hemodynamically stable. Assume wide-complex, regular tachyarrhythmias in WPW syndrome are conducting down the accessory pathway and treat with synchronized cardioversion, although again procainamide or amiodarone is often tried if hemodynamically stable. Cardiology consultation is always appropriate. Ablation of accessory pathways plays an important role as a permanent solution in recurrent tachyarrhythmias with WPW syndrome.

233 i. Nummular dermatitis (aka nummular eczema), characterized by round-to-oval erythematous plaques most commonly found on the extremities, trunk, and anywhere but the face. Lesions often begin as papules, which then coalesce into scaly plaques. Allergy and irritant factors tend to cause exacerbations, particularly contact sensitivity to clothes, metal jewelry, or occupational exposures.

ii. Recognition and elimination of allergic and irritant factors is necessary. Cool baths, with minimal soap use, and skin moisturizers (e.g. petroleum jelly) may help rehydrate the skin. Topical corticosteroids are helpful. Tar preparations and topical immunomodulators (e.g. tacrolimus) also reduce inflammation. Oral antihistamines may reduce itching and improve sleep. Oral antibiotics may be necessary in cases with secondary infection.

234 A 19-year-old female had daily stabbing headaches (her exact words) since being involved in an altercation at a bar about 1 year ago. She was struck in the head at that time with what she thought was a glass and passed out. She awoke with a cut on her head, but never sought medical attention. Any thoughts after viewing this radiograph (234a)?

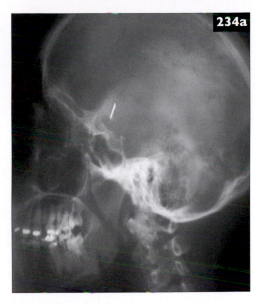

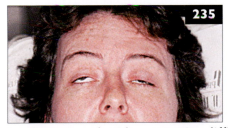

235 A 32-year-old female presented with progressive difficulty speaking and swallowing over the past few weeks, along with intermittent double vision and general fatigue (235). She was not taking any medications and had no previous medical problems.
i. What are the differential diagnoses with these findings?
ii. How would you confirm the diagnosis?
iii. How is this condition treated?

234 It looks like a simple piece of retained metal, which might be irritating the scalp and causing local pain. An anterior–posterior radiograph was obtained to further characterize the foreign body (234b). That film is stunning, as it clearly shows a broken knife blade (arrow) deeply embedded in the brain. The patient required a craniotomy with careful neurosurgical technique to remove this surprising headache trigger. Just another reason to drink a bit less alcohol!

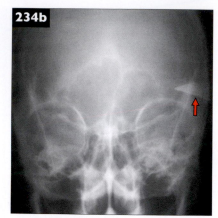

235 i. Myasthenia gravis (MG) is the most common disorder of neuromuscular transmission. Consider botulism (more rapid, progressive time course) or certain medications (e.g. penicillamine, statins). Brainstem pathology and disorders that compress multiple cranial nerves present similarly. The Miller Fisher variant of Guillain–Barré syndrome may demonstrate oculopharyngeal weakness, as may oculopharyngeal muscular dystrophy. Organophosphate intoxication and mitochondrial disorders with ophthalmoplegia are other possibilities. Factitious disorders must be considered.

ii. MG is an autoimmune disorder with an annual incidence about 2–4 per million and most common in women <40 or men >60 years old. Weakness is due to circulating acetylcholine receptor antibodies affecting mostly postsynaptic neuromuscular junctions. Patients have muscle fatigue with repetitive activity, with eyes and facial muscles most affected. Limb and neck muscles may also be involved, as well as muscles of respiration. MG has a fluctuating course. Physical examination may elicit muscle fatigue by repetitive eye movements or multiple limb exercises. IV edrophonium, a short-acting acetylcholinesterase inhibitor, temporarily increases muscle strength in MG and is used by experienced consultants to aid diagnosis. Electromyography is sensitive, showing a decremental response to repetitive stimulation. Chest radiography or CT may reveal an enlarged thymus. Serologic tests reveal acetylcholine receptor antibodies in 80–95%, but less commonly with only ocular MG. Pulmonary function studies quantitate respiratory fatigue.

iii. Primary treatments are cholinesterase inhibitors (e.g. pyridostigmine) and immunosuppressive agents (e.g. prednisone, cyclosporine). Plasmapheresis, as well as IV immunoglobulins, may give temporary improvement in severe MG. Intubation with ventilation may be necessary in respiratory failure. Thymoma should be resected, and even removal of a normal thymus may help.

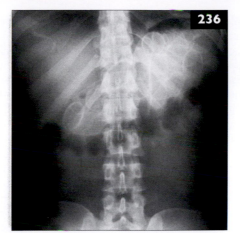

236 A 27-year-old male presented with recurrent vomiting and constipation.
i. What does this abdominal radiograph suggest is the problem (236)?
ii. How is this managed?

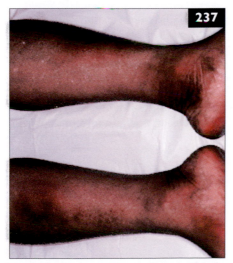

237 A 31-year-old female had a recent sore throat. She developed these painful nodules on her shins a few days after starting an unknown antibiotic (237).
i. What do you think is the problem?
ii. What are likely causes?
iii. How should she be treated?

236 i. The radiograph shows a large number of machine-wrapped packets of drugs, which had been concealed for international smuggling by this patient (often referred to as a body packer, courier, or mule). Occasionally, a body packer may have drugs in latex balloons as simple as condoms or fingers of gloves, which often leak or rupture in the intestinal tract or vagina, resulting in massive drug overdose. Typically, diagnosis is by abdominal radiography, with heroin-filled balloons very hypodense, cocaine about stool density, and hashish more radiopaque than stool. (Heroin was in these.) Patients often consume excessive amounts of antispasmodics to prevent passage during transport, which may lead to intestinal obstruction and/or recurrent vomiting.

ii. Besides the complex legal issues, usually it is only necessary to allow the packets to pass naturally. Oil-based laxatives may weaken the packaging and thus cause leakage, which should be avoided. Whole bowel irrigation with oral polyethylene glycol has been reported to hasten packet removal. With symptomatic packet rupture or intestinal obstruction, surgical removal may be necessary.

237 i. Erythema nodosum, an acute, nodular, erythematous eruption that usually presents on extensor surfaces of lower extremities. It is most common in young adults. The eruptive phase begins with fever, arthralgias, and generalized body aches.

ii. Erythema nodosum is a delayed hypersensitivity reaction due to an assortment of antigens. Various bacterial infections (particularly *Streptococcus*), fungal causes, drugs, inflammatory bowel diseases, rheumatologic disorders, lymphomas, sarcoidosis, and pregnancy are likely causes. Identification is usually clinical and biopsy is reserved for diagnostically difficult cases. Work-up is only necessary if the etiology is not obvious.

iii. Treatment is based on management of the underlying disease or withdrawal of precipitating medications. Spontaneous regression generally occurs and NSAIDs are usually all that are needed for symptomatic relief. Corticosteroids are effective, but are often not necessary. Recurrence is common, particularly if the underlying cause is not resolved.

238 A 32-year-old male developed sudden eye pain while he was hammering a jammed metal gear at work about 8 hours ago. He felt something in his right eye, but he wiped it out. He presented with mild right eye pain and some blurred vision. Examination showed only a small subconjunctival hemorrhage over the inferior eye sclera on the right. Visual acuity was decreased in the right eye.

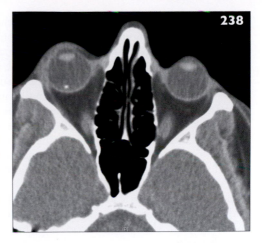

i. What does this CT image suggest is going on here (238)?
ii. How should he be managed?

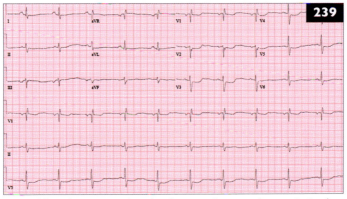

239 A 71-year-old male presented with 2 hours of severe chest pain in the precordial region, with shortness of breath and nausea. BP was 112/70 mmHg (14.9/9.3 kPa), P 60 bpm, and RR 24/min.
i. Does he meet the criteria for immediate coronary revascularization (239)?
ii. What clinical changes might prompt further intervention?

238 i. There is a visible foreign body in the posterior globe of his right eye. Intraocular foreign bodies vary in size and shape, with about 90% metallic. The most important prognostic factor is the damage occurring with injury. The most common causative event is hammering metal, and most intraocular foreign bodies come to rest in the posterior segment. A careful examination of both eyes, including visual acuities, is important. Occasionally, as in this case, minimal evidence of external eye injury occurs despite eye globe penetration. This is particularly a problem with delayed presentations. Simple radiographs are usually diagnostic, although CT is the imaging modality of choice for intraocular foreign body localization in complex cases. Ultrasound has also been used successfully. Avoid MRI if the foreign body could be ferromagnetic.

ii. Systemic and topical antibiotics should be initiated before surgical intervention. Topical corticosteroids also help to minimize inflammation. Prompt ophthalmologic evaluation is important, as intraocular foreign body removal is almost always necessary and should be done promptly in wounds with a high risk of endophthalmitis.

239 i. This patient has sinus bradycardia at about 60 bpm with 1–2 mm of ST depression in leads V_1–V_5. In this clinical setting the patient has an acute coronary syndrome, most likely non-STEMI. Comparison with previous ECGs, if available, is useful to confirm that these changes are new. Measurement of serial cardiac markers will likely confirm infarction.

ii. Thrombolytic therapy has never been shown to reduce morbidity or mortality in non-STEMI, and it indeed may worsen outcomes. Emergency percutaneous intervention is clearly indicated in STEMI, but its use in non-STEMI is more complex. Risk stratification is necessary for stable non-STEMI patients, as early mortality is actually increased with percutaneous intervention in low-risk patients. Continued unstable vital signs, significant arrhythmias, ongoing chest pain unresponsive to medical therapy, and serial increases of cardiac biomarkers are clear indications for prompt percutaneous intervention. Increased age, diabetes mellitus, prior myocardial infarction, hypertension, high or low body mass index, elevated cardiac biomarkers, recurrent rest angina, cardiac arrest at admission, and continued ST segment deviation are among the risk factors that together help define those patients likely to benefit from early percutaneous intervention in stable non-STEMI.

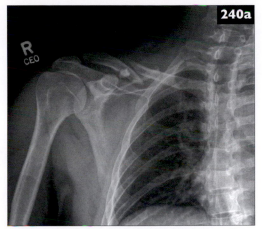

240 A 32-year-old male was involved in a motor vehicle collision and complained of severe pain when he moved his right shoulder.
i. What is the problem (240a)?
ii. How should this be managed?

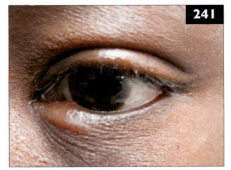

241 A 36-year-old female presented with 2 days of eye pain and lower lid swelling (241).
i. What is the problem?
ii. How should it be treated?

240 i. A comminuted mid-shaft clavicle (or collarbone) fracture, the second most commonly broken bone in the body (nasal bone is number one). About 80% are middle-third fractures, with 15% distal third. Most fractures occur proximal to the coracoclavicular ligament, with the proximal fragment displaced upwards by the sternocleido-

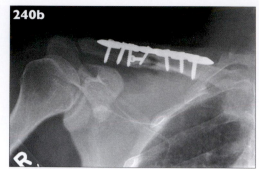

mastoid muscle. Usual mechanism of injury in clavicle fracture is force applied to the lateral shoulder by a fall or motor vehicle collision. Diagnosis is usually clinical by palpation of local swelling, tenderness, and crepitus, with confirmation by simple radiographs. CT may help in complex cases. Associated neurovascular injuries are rare, but pneumothorax can occur.

ii. Pain control is important. Although a figure-of-eight clavicle splint has traditionally been employed, recent studies show more pain using this method without any improvement in clinical outcome when compared with management using a simple arm sling. Although mid-clavicular fractures have been treated conservatively, recent studies show improved functional outcome, with less malunion and nonunion, using operative management of displaced fractures, particularly those with 2 cm or more of initial shortening (**240b**).

241 i. Hordeolum, a common localized infection of either the glands of Zeis (stye) or, less commonly, the meibomian glands (internal hordeolum). Stasis of secretions leads to secondary infection, usually by *Staphylococcus aureus*. Hordeolum should not be confused with chalazion, a chronic lipogranulomatous inflammation of these glands that is not infectious. Hordeolum is basically a focal abscess, which presents with an erythematous, painful, swollen nodule in the eyelid. Diagnosis is by clinical recognition.

ii. Hordeolum is a self-limiting infection that usually responds to warm compresses applied for 10–15 minutes several times a day. Topical antibiotic ointment may be useful if there is associated blepharoconjunctivitis. Systemic antibiotics may be indicated if there is preseptal cellulitis. Surgical drainage under local anesthesia is indicated for a large hordeolum or if refractory to standard therapy.

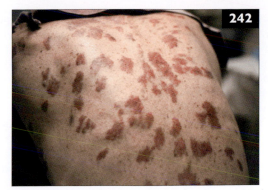

242 A 34-year-old homosexual male had multiple bruises on his back, which were bumpy and had come up over several weeks (242).
i. What is this condition?
ii. How should it be evaluated and treated?

243 A 31-year-old male fell approximately 6 meters (20 feet) off scaffolding and landed on his out-stretched arm. After initial management of a left shoulder dislocation, it was noted his left wrist was swollen and tender.
i. What does this wrist radiograph show (243)?
ii. What treatment is required?

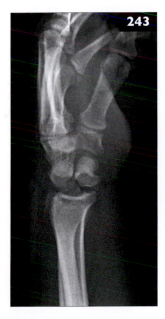

242 i. Extensive Kaposi's sarcoma, a malignancy caused by human herpesvirus 8 (aka Kaposi's sarcoma-associated herpesvirus). Four forms are described: classic, an indolent disease among elderly men usually of Mediterranean origin; endemic, described in young Africans mainly from sub-Saharan Africa and unrelated to HIV infection; immunosuppression-associated, especially with calcineurin inhibitor (e.g. cyclosporine) use; and AIDS-associated in HIV-infected individuals. Kaposi's sarcoma is an AIDS-defining illness and the presenting problem in many HIV patients. Kaposi's sarcoma typically is found in the skin as papules and nodules that may be red, purple, brown, or even black. Spread to the gastrointestinal and/or respiratory tract is common. Kaposi's sarcoma is actually not a sarcoma, but a cancer of lymphatic endothelium that forms vascular channels and resulting in its characteristic appearance.

ii. A definitive diagnosis can only be made by biopsy, which shows characteristic spindle cells. HIV status should be defined. Kaposi's sarcoma is not curable, but palliation may add years of life. Reduction of immunosuppressive medications should be accomplished, if possible. HAART therapy in HIV patients leads to Kaposi's sarcoma remission in at least 40%. Radiation therapy or cryosurgery may be helpful for local lesions. Multiple chemotherapeutic and immunotherapeutic agents are effective in Kaposi's sarcoma.

243 i. Wrist injuries are common and frequently missed in polysystem trauma. In this lateral radiograph, the kidney bean-shaped lunate is spilled and displaced volar from its normal position between the distal radius and capitate. A small dorsal avulsion fracture of the distal radius is also present. The mechanism of lunate dislocation is usually a fall with hyperextension of an outstretched hand. The lunate normally sits with its concave surface as the base for the capitate. Associated ligamentous disruptions and occasional neurovascular compromise are the main acute problems, with chronic wrist pain and arthritis potential long-term issues.

ii. Closed reduction can be attempted under adequate procedural sedation, but even successful lunate repositioning will usually need later surgery for ligament repair. Open reduction of lunate dislocation is frequently necessary, and repair of associated injuries can be done at that time.

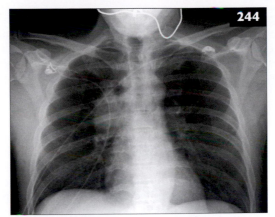

244 A 63-year-old male presented with increased facial swelling and morning headaches over the past few days.
i. What is the likely diagnosis based on this chest radiograph (**244**)?
ii. How should it be managed?

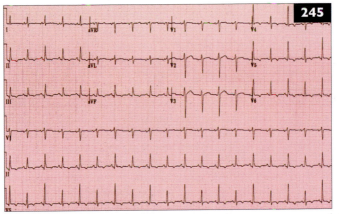

245 A 53-year-old male presented with progressive dyspnea over several days, with no known prior medical problems other than alcohol abuse.
i. What does the ECG suggest (**245**)?
ii. How would you confirm the diagnosis?

244 i. This large superior mediastinal mass, along with associated symptoms, suggests superior vena cava (SVC) syndrome. This is usually caused by primary lung malignancy (small cell lung cancer in two-thirds); Hodgkin's lymphoma and a few others cause most of the rest. Nonmalignant causes of SVC syndrome are numerous, particularly catheter-related thrombosis and infectious etiologies (e.g. tuberculosis). Dyspnea is the most common symptom, but facial and upper extremity swelling, headache, difficulty swallowing, cough, hoarseness, and stridor can occur. Diagnosis is clinical, with chest radiographs showing superior mediastinal or right upper lobe mass in most with a malignant cause. Chest CT is usually confirmatory, as is MRI and contrast venography.

ii. Most patients with malignant SVC syndrome lack an initial etiologic diagnosis. Except in true emergencies (e.g. altered mental status due to cerebral edema), primary diagnosis should be obtained before treatment. Sputum cytology, bronchoscopy, mediastinoscopy, node biopsy, and thoracotomy have increasing diagnositic success, in about that order. Treatment is etiologic. Head elevation and supplemental oxygen may help, with corticosteroids used to relieve cerebral or laryngeal edema. Radiation therapy is effective for most patients. Chemotherapy is useful in selective tumors, particularly small cell lung cancer and lymphomas. Vena cava stenting has palliative utility in many patients. Thrombolytics or anti-coagulation with catheter removal may be successful with SVC thrombosis.

245 i. The ECG shows sinus tachycardia with ventricular rate approximately 120 bpm. There is electrical alternans, defined as alternate beat variation in direction, amplitude, or duration of any component of the ECG waveform. It is usually due to the heart swinging anterior and posterior with each heartbeat in a bag of pericardial fluid. Electrical alternans is usually only seen with fairly large pericardial effusions. These may be asymptomatic or may compress the heart as pressure rises in the pericardial sac. Total electrical alternans (P, QRS, and T wave) frequently suggests pericardial tamponade, but this is only seen in 5–10% of patients with this problem. Electrical alternans due to heart movement has also been reported in hypertrophic cardiomyopathy.

ii. Ultrasound or echocardiography can rapidly confirm pericardial effusion. Diastolic collapse of the right atrium and paradoxical ventricular septal shift are highly suggestive of pericardial tamponade. Percutaneous or surgical drainage of the pericardium, along with volume resuscitation, is the emergency intervention of choice for hemodynamically significant pericardial tamponade.

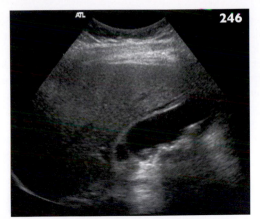

246 A 47-year-old male presented with recurrent episodes of vomiting and right upper abdominal pain, usually after meals. The pain had been continuous all day.
i. What does this ultrasound image demonstrate (246)?
ii. How should the patient be managed?

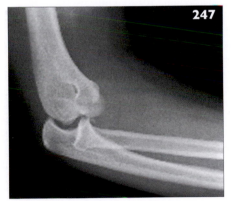

247 A 27-year-old patient fell on her outstretched hand and had immediate severe pain in the elbow.
i. What is the diagnosis (247)?
ii. How is this managed?

246 i. The image shows the liver and a longitudinal view of the gallbladder. The gallbladder is enlarged, with multiple gallstones along with a large amount of posterior acoustic shadowing. Importantly, a small amount of anterior pericholecystic fluid is seen, suggesting acute cholecystitis. Gallbladder wall thickening (>4 mm) and a sonographic Murphy's sign (exacerbation of pain by pressing the probe directly over the gallbladder) are also seen in acute cholecystitis. Additional views are necessary to look for dilation of the common bile duct (>6 mm), which is suggestive of choledocholithiasis.

ii. There is ultrasound evidence of cholecystitis, therefore the patient needs broad-spectrum antibiotics to cover gram-negative organisms in particular. CBC, liver enzymes, and amylase or lipase levels are indicated. Early surgical consultation is necessary to evaluate for possible cholecystectomy.

247 i. Posterior elbow dislocation. Considerable force is required to dislocate the elbow joint, and a third will have associated fracture. Elbow dislocation without fracture is called simple, and with fracture is called complex. Anterior elbow dislocation is less common, typically caused by a posterior elbow blow. Elbow dislocation is painful, usually presenting with joint swelling and limited range of motion. Posterior elbow dislocation presents in flexion with an exaggerated olecranon prominence, while anterior dislocation presents with elbow hyperextension, forearm shortening, and supination. Associated brachial artery and/or median nerve injuries are more common with anterior elbow dislocation. Plain radiographs are usually adequate for diagnosis.

ii. Prehospital management should include splinting in position and pain management. In the hospital, simple elbow dislocation should be promptly reduced, particularly if there is vascular compromise, in which case even complex dislocation should have reduction attempted. Sedation and analgesia are required. The traditional traction reduction technique, as well as a prone method, has been described. Multiple approaches may be necessary for reduction. All successful elbow reductions should be placed in a posterior splint at 70–90° of flexion, with the forearm neutral to pronation and supination. Complex elbow dislocations often require surgical reduction and fixation. Delayed vascular compromise due to occult brachial artery injury is a dreaded complication, so observe patients for several hours after reduction. Vascular injury should prompt immediate appropriate consultation, as should median or ulnar nerve dysfunction.

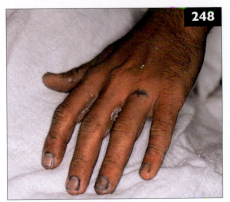

248 A 27-year-old male presented with severe bilateral hand pain, which had become progressively more severe over the past 24 hours. He worked at a car detailing (intensive cleaning) shop and spent much of yesterday cleaning chrome with special chemicals.
i. What do the history and these hand findings suggest (**248**)?
ii. How should it be evaluated and treated?

249 A 22-year-old female had an arteriovenous fistula placed at her right antecubital fossa 6 days ago. She presented with right upper extremity swelling that was mildly painful. She had a strong thrill at the fistula site.
i. What does this photograph suggest (**249**)?
ii. What evaluation is indicated?

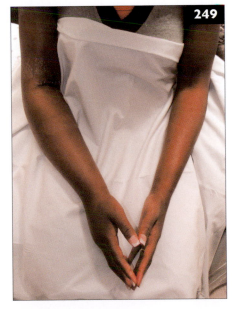

251

248 i. Chrome cleaner often contains hydrofluoric acid. This strong acid may have delayed onset of significant burns in dilute concentrations because of the tendency for deep skin penetration before dissociation. It may be absorbed dermally or inhalationally. Most exposures are to small areas such as fingers. Injury is due to acid corrosion, as well as deep penetration of fluoride ion. Hydrofluoric acid burns present with severe pain to involved skin despite little apparent injury. Dilute solutions (<10%) may delay presentations for several hours, while concentrated solutions (>20%) produce prompt classic burn findings of erythema, blistering, and skin necrosis. Fluoride ions form insoluble salts with magnesium and calcium. Severe exposures may cause tetany as well as cardiac arrhythmias.

ii. Obtain the exact product name or container if possible. Understanding the concentration of hydrofluoric acid used, other chemicals in the solution, as well as time, surface area, and duration of exposure is important. Check electrolytes, including calcium and magnesium. Obtain an ECG, looking for prolonged QT interval (hypocalcemia, hypomagnesemia), or evidence of hyperkalemia in severe cases. Start treatment of exposure with skin decontamination, using copious water to all exposed skin. Monitor cardiac rhythm and give IV calcium gluconate or chloride if there is evidence of severe hypocalcemia. Soak exposed skin in 2.5% calcium gluconate gel (one volume 10% calcium gluconate to three volumes of water soluble lubricant). Rarely, subcutaneous, IV, or intra-arterial injections of calcium gluconate are necessary for ongoing burns unresponsive to topical therapy.

249 i. Complications of arteriovenous fistula for hemodialysis vascular access are common. Simple edema due to resultant venous hypertension is frequent, will resolve with time, and improves more rapidly with extremity elevation. Hematomas are common at the surgical site, as are aneurysms and pseudoaneurysms. Occasionally, arterial ischemia occurs due to a steal syndrome caused by excessive arteriovenous shunting, which presents with distal extremity pain along with cyanosis or pallor of the fingers. Venous stenosis and/or thrombosis may also occur and create distal extremity edema.

ii. Ultrasound is excellent in evaluation of arteriovenous fistulas, both early and late. As this patient has a palpable thrill at the fistula site and no evidence of ischemia, simple arm elevation may be all that is necessary. Discussion with the vascular surgeon who created the arteriovenous fistula is appropriate.

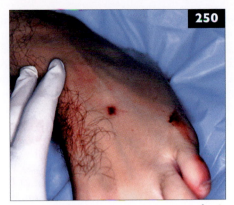

250 A 37-year-old male had a recent upper respiratory infection and presented with severe headache, fever (39.7°C), and diffuse myalgias. Physical examination revealed a supple neck, normal neurologic examination, and this rash (250).
i. What is the differential diagnosis in this situation?
ii. How should the patient be managed?

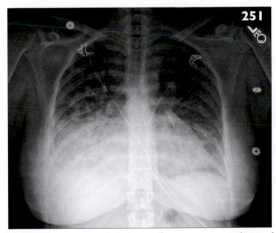

251 A 27-year-old female presented 5 days after an uncomplicated vaginal delivery with 2 days of increasing shortness of breath and nonproductive cough. BP was 164/104 mmHg (21.9/13.9 kPa) with P 152 bpm, RR 28/min, and T 36.6°C.
i. What does this chest radiograph suggest is the proper diagnosis (251)?
ii. What treatment is indicated?

250 i. This is a purpuric rash, usually due to vessel inflammation from vasculitis, collagen vascular disease, infection, or drug reaction. Thrombocytopenia due to various causes may also cause purpura. Although purpura with fever may be caused by any of these, infection is most likely. Many infectious agents can cause purpuric rash, but rickettsial disease, malaria, staphylococci, and gram-negative agents, including meningococci, are most common. In this patient with a purpuric rash and fever with severe headache, meningitis must be considered, particularly secondary to *Neisseria meningitidis*.

ii. Immediate evaluation for infection with concomitant antibiotic therapy is important. CBC, blood cultures, coagulation studies, and a urinalysis should be done. Lumbar puncture is indicated here, as meningococcal meningitis in particular may have a supple neck early in the illness. PCR testing of CSF fluid may rapidly confirm meningococcal or other bacterial causes of meningitis. Penicillin remains the antibiotic of choice for meningococcemia, but broad-spectrum coverage may be indicated until definitive confirmation of the offending organism.

251 i. Peripartum cardiomyopathy (PPCM) with significant heart failure. PPCM is a rare form of dilated cardiomyopathy that occurs in the last month of pregnancy to as late as 6 months postpartum. It has an incidence of 1 in 3,000–4,000 live births. Risk factors include obesity, hypertension, age >30 years, African-American race, multiple pregnancies, and pre-eclampsia. Although nutritional, autoimmune, and impaired cardiac microvascular perfusion are proposed etiologies, recent research suggests increased peripartum oxidative stress leads to proteolytic cleavage of prolactin to a subform with antiangiogenic, proinflammatory, and proapoptotic factors. Typical presentations are those of systolic dysfunction with low ejection fraction, often with pulmonary edema, evidence of tissue hypoperfusion, and occasionally with vascular emboli.

ii. Similar to conventional therapy for heart failure: oxygen therapy if hypoxic, vasodilators (e.g. angiotensin-converting enzyme inhibitors), diuretics, cardiac glycosides, and anticoagulation for very low ejection fraction patients. Severe failure may require aggressive airway intervention and pressor therapy. Beta blockers may be added when overt heart failure has been stabilized. Blockade of prolactin by bromocriptine, a dopamine D2 receptor agonist, prevented PPCM in an experimental model and helped in a small pilot trial of patients with PPCM. Recent studies show survival from PPCM is up to 98%, and at least 50% recover normal systolic function. Recurrence rate of PPCM is at least 20% with subsequent pregnancy.

Further reading

Case 1

Erling BF, Perron AD, Brady WJ (2004) Disagreement in the interpretation of electrocardiographic ST segment elevation: a source of error for emergency physicians? *Am J Emerg Med* **22**:65–70.

Smith SW (2006) ST segment elevation differs depending on the method of measurement. *Acad Emerg Med* **13**:406–412.

Case 2

Michelson JD (2003) Ankle fractures resulting from rotational injuries. *J Am Acad Orthop Surg* **11**:403–412.

Ng A, Barnes ES (2009) Management of complications of open reduction and internal fixation of ankle fractures. *Clin Podiatr Med Surg* **26**:105–125.

Case 3

Kauvar DS, Wade CE (2005) The epidemiology and modern management of traumatic hemorrhage: US and international perspectives. *Crit Care* **9(Suppl 5)**:S1–9.

Lienhart HG, Lindner KH, Wenzel V (2008) Developing alternative strategies for the treatment of traumatic haemorrhagic shock. *Curr Opin Crit Care* **14**:247–253.

Case 4

Ahrens T, Sona C (2003) Capnography application in acute and critical care. *AACN Clin Issues* **14**:123–132.

Kupnik D, Skok P (2007) Capnometry in the prehospital setting: are we using its potential? *Emerg Med J* **24**:614–617

Case 5

Feller L, Lemmer J (2008) Necrotizing periodontal diseases in HIV-seropositive subjects: pathogenic mechanisms. *J Intl Acad Periodontol* **10**:10–15.

Wade DN, Kerns DG (1998) Acute necrotizing ulcerative gingivitis-periodontitis: a literature review. *Mil Med* **163**:337–342.

Case 6

Centor RM, Allison JJ, Cohen SJ (2007) Pharyngitis management: defining the controversy. *J Gen Intern Med* **22**:127–130.

Del Mar CB, Glasziou PP, Spinks AB (2006) Antibiotics for sore throat. *Cochrane Database Syst Rev* **Oct 18**:CD000023.

Case 7

Maskill JD, Bohay DR, Anderson JG (2005) Calcaneus fractures: a review article. *Foot Ankle Clin* **10**:463–489.

Swanson SA, Clare MP, Sanders RW (2008) Management of intra-articular fractures of the calcaneus. *Foot Ankle Clin* **13**:659–678.

Case 8

Kraut JA, Kurtz I (2008) Toxic alcohol ingestions: clinical features, diagnosis, and management. *Clin J Am Soc Nephrol* **3**:208–225.

Leth PM, Gregersen M (2005) Ethylene glycol poisoning. *Forensic Sci Int* **155**:179–184.

Case 9

Dirschl DR, Dawson PA (2004) Injury severity assessment in tibial plateau fractures. *Clin Orthop Rel Res* **423**:85–92.

Musahl V, Tarkin I, Kobbe P *et al.* (2009) New trends and techniques in open reduction and internal fixation of fractures of the tibial plateau. *J Bone Joint Surg Br* **91**:426–433.

Case 10
Mokhlesi B, Garimella PS, Joffe A *et al.* (2004) Street drug abuse leading to critical illness. *Intens Care Med* **30**:1526–1536.

Vroegop MP, Franssen EJ, van der Voort PH *et al.* (2009) The emergency care of cocaine intoxications. *Neth J Med* **67**:122–126.

Case 11
Gilbert SC (2007) Management and prevention of recurrent herpes labialis in immunocompetent patients. *Herpes* **14**:56–61.

Opstelten W, Neven AK, Eekhof J (2008) Treatment and prevention of herpes labialis. *Can Fam Physician* **54**:1683–1687.

Case 12
Fitzgerald JE, Fitzgerald LA, Anderson FE *et al.* (2009) The changing nature of rectus sheath haematoma: case series and literature review. *Int J Surg* **7**:150–154.

Osinbowale O, Bartholomew JR (2008) Rectus sheath hematoma. *Vasc Med* **13**:275–279.

Case 13
Edlich RF, Farinholt HM, Winters KL *et al.* (2005) Modern concepts of treatment and prevention of electrical burns. *J Long-Term Eff Med* **15**:511–532.

Koumbourlis AC (2002) Electrical injuries. *Crit Care Med* **30(11 Suppl)**:S424–430.

Case 14
Buylaert WA (2000) Coma induced by intoxication. *Acta Neurol Belg* **100**:221–224.

Cook S, Moeschler O, Michaud K *et al.* (1998) Acute opiate overdose: characteristics of 190 consecutive cases. *Addiction* **93**:1559–1565.

Case 15
Haan JM, Bochicchio GV, Kramer N *et al.* (2005) Nonoperative management of blunt splenic injury: a 5-year experience. *J Trauma* **58**:492–498.

Raikhlin A, Baerlocher MO, Asch MR *et al.* (2008) Imaging and transcatheter arterial embolization for traumatic splenic injuries: review of the literature. *Can J Surg* **51**:464–472.

Case 16
Budzikowski AS, Uyguanco E, Gunsburg MY *et al.* (2008) Twisting until it breaks: a rare cause of ICD lead failure. *Cardiol J* **15**:558–560.

Morin DP, Iwai S (2010) Iatrogenic Twiddler's syndrome. *J Interv Card Electr* **29**:135–137.

Case 17
Lafrance JP, Rahme E, Lelorier J *et al.* (2008) Vascular access-related infections: definitions, incidence rates, and risk factors. *Am J Kidney Dis* **52**:982–993.

Padberg FT Jr, Calligaro KD, Sidawy AN (2008) Complications of arteriovenous hemodialysis access: recognition and management. *J Vasc Surg* **48(5 Suppl)**:55S–80S.

Case 18
Gavignet B, Piarroux R, Aubin F *et al.* (2008) Cutaneous manifestations of human toxocariasis. *J Am Acad Dermatol* **59**:1031–1042.

Heukelbach J, Feldmeier H (2008) Epidemiological and clinical characteristics of hookworm-related cutaneous larva migrans. *Lancet Infect Dis* **8**:302–309.

Case 19
Mark BJ, Slavin RG (2006) Allergic contact dermatitis. *Med Clin North Am* 90:169–185.
Nosbaum A, Vocanson M, Rozieres A *et al.* (2009) Allergic and irritant contact dermatitis. *Eur J Dermatol* 19:325–332.

Case 20
Chin SH, Vedder NB (2008) MOC-PSSM CME article: metacarpal fractures. *Plast Reconstr Surg* 121(1 Suppl):1–13.
Henry MH (2008) Fractures of the proximal phalanx and metacarpals in the hand: preferred methods of stabilization. *J Am Acad Orthop Surg* 16:586–595.

Case 21
Brook I (2009) The bacteriology of salivary gland infections. *Oral Maxillofac Surg Clin North Am* 21:269–274.
Cascarini L, McGurk M (2009) Epidemiology of salivary gland infections. *Oral Maxillofac Surg Clin North Am* 21:353–357.

Case 22
Ma G, Brady WJ, Pollack M *et al.* (2001) Electrocardiographic manifestations: digitalis toxicity. *J Emerg Med* 20:145–152.
Vivo RP, Krim SR, Perez J *et al.* (2008) Digoxin: current use and approach to toxicity. *Am J Med Sci* 336:423–428.

Case 23
Diringer MN (2009) Management of aneurysmal subarachnoid hemorrhage. *Crit Care Med* 37:432–440.
Wijdicks EF, Kallmes DF, Manno EM *et al.* (2005) Subarachnoid hemorrhage: neurointensive care and aneurysm repair. *Mayo Clin Proc* 80:550–559.

Case 24
Look KM, Look RM (1997) Skin scraping, cupping, and moxibustion that may mimic physical abuse. *J Forensic Sci* 42:103–105.

Wong HC, Wong JK, Wong NY (1999) Signs of physical abuse or evidence of moxibustion, cupping or coining? *Can Med Assoc J* 160:785–786.

Case 25
Eccleston K, Collins L, Higgins SP *et al.* (2008) Primary syphilis. *Int J STD AIDS* 19:145–151.
Lautenschlager S (2006) Diagnosis of syphilis: clinical and laboratory problems. *J Dtsch Dermatol Ges* 4:1058–1075.

Case 26
Temmerman W, Dhondt A, Vandewoude K (1999) Acute isoniazid intoxication: seizures, acidosis and coma. *Acta Clinica Belgica* 54:211–216.
Topcu I, Yentur EA, Kefi A *et al.* (2005) Seizures, metabolic acidosis and coma resulting from acute isoniazid intoxication. *Anaesth Intens Care* 33:518–520.

Case 27
Chen SC, Lee CC, Liu YP *et al.* (2005) Ultrasound may decrease the emergency surgery rate of incarcerated inguinal hernia. *Scand J Gastroenterol* 40:721–724.
Deeba S, Purkayastha S, Paraskevas P *et al.* (2009) Laparoscopic approach to incarcerated and strangulated inguinal hernias. *J Soc Lap Surg* 13:327–331.

Case 28
Bathala EA, Bancroft LW, Ortiguera CJ *et al.* (2007) Radiologic case study: segond fracture. *Orthopedics* 30:689, 797–798.
Gottsegen CJ, Eyer BA, White EA *et al.* (2008) Avulsion fractures of the knee: imaging findings and clinical significance. *Radiographics* 28:1755–1770.

Case 29

Peretz A, Guillaume MP, Casper-Velu L (2002) Uveitis management: a multidisciplinary approach to assess systemic involvement and side effects of treatments. *Acta Clinica Belgica* 57:142–147.

Ramsay A, Lightman S (2001) Hypopyon uveitis. *Surv Ophthalmol* 46:1–18.

Case 30

Pirronti T, Macis G, Meduri A *et al.* (1996) Chest radiograph in pulmonary embolism. *Rays* 21:352–362.

Srivastava SD, Eagleton MJ, Greenfield LJ (2004) Diagnosis of pulmonary embolism with various imaging modalities. *Sem Vasc Surg* 17:173–180.

Case 31

Chui J, Di Girolamo N, Wakefield D *et al.* (2008) The pathogenesis of pterygium: current concepts and their therapeutic implications. *Ocul Surf* 6:24–43.

Detorakis ET, Spandidos DA (2009) Pathogenetic mechanisms and treatment options for ophthalmic pterygium: trends and perspectives. *Int J Mol Med* 23:439–447.

Case 32

Li Q, Chen N, Yang J *et al.* (2009) Antiviral treatment for preventing postherpetic neuralgia. *Cochrane Database Syst Rev* Apr 15:CD006866.

Sampathkumar P, Drage LA, Martin DP (2009) Herpes zoster (shingles) and postherpetic neuralgia. *Mayo Clin Proc* 84:274–280.

Case 33

Ash-Bernal R, Wise R, Wright SM (2004) Acquired methemoglobinemia: a retrospective series of 138 cases at 2 teaching hospitals. *Medicine* 83:265–273.

do Nascimento TS, Pereira RO, de Mello HL (2008) Methemoglobinemia: from diagnosis to treatment. *Rev Bras Anestesiol* 58:651–664.

Case 34

Kalainov DM, Hoepfner PE, Hartigan BJ *et al.* (2005) Nonsurgical treatment of closed mallet finger fractures. *J Hand Surg* 30:580–586.

Leinberry C (2009) Mallet finger injuries. *J Hand Surg* 34:1715–1717.

Case 35

Byrnes MC, Mazuski JE (2009) Antimicrobial therapy for acute colonic diverticulitis. *Surg Infect* 10:143–154.

Touzios JG, Dozois EJ (2009) Diverticulosis and acute diverticulitis. *Gastroenterol Clin North Am* 38:513–525.

Case 36

Buck ML, Wiggins BS, Sesler JM (2007) Intraosseous drug administration in children and adults during cardiopulmonary resuscitation. *Ann Pharmacother* 41:1679–1686.

Von Hoff DD, Kuhn JG, Burris HA 3rd *et al.* (2008) Does intraosseous equal intravenous? A pharmacokinetic study. *Am J Emerg Med* 26:31–38.

Case 37

Alkaabi JM, Mushtaq A, Al-Maskari FN *et al.* (2010) Hypokalemic periodic paralysis: a case series, review of the literature and update of management. *Eur J Emerg Med* 17:45–47.

Finsterer J (2008) Primary periodic paralyses. *Acta Neurol Scand* 117:145–158.

Case 38

Veien NK (2009) Acute and recurrent vesicular hand dermatitis. *Dermatol Clin* 27:337–353.

Wollina U (2008) Pompholyx: what's new? *Expert Opin Investig Drugs* 17:897–904.

Case 39

Isbister GK, Graudins A, White J *et al.* (2003) Antivenom treatment in arachnidism. *J Toxicol Clin Toxic* 41:291–300.

Vetter RS, Isbister GK (2008) Medical aspects of spider bites. *Ann Rev Entomol* **53**:409–429.

Case 40
Herbella FA, Mudo M, Delmonti C *et al.* (2001) 'Raccoon eyes' (periorbital haematoma) as a sign of skull base fracture. *Injury* **32**:745–747.
Pretto Flores L, De Almeida CS, Casulari LA (2000) Positive predictive values of selected clinical signs associated with skull base fractures. *J Neurosurg Sci* **44**:77–82.

Case 41
Dundas B, Harris M, Narasimhan M (2007) Psychogenic polydipsia review: etiology, differential, and treatment. *Curr Psychiatry Rep* **9**:236–241.
Reddy P, Mooradian AD (2009) Diagnosis and management of hyponatraemia in hospitalised patients. *Int J Clin Pract* **63**:1494–1508.

Case 42
Patlas M, Farkas A, Fisher D *et al.* (2001) Ultrasound vs CT for the detection of ureteric stones in patients with renal colic. *Brit J Radiol* **74**:901–904.
Singh A, Alter HJ, Littlepage A (2007) A systematic review of medical therapy to facilitate passage of ureteral calculi. *Ann Emerg Med* **50**:552–563.

Case 43
Jana N, Santra D, Das D *et al.* (2008) Nonobstetric lower genital tract injuries in rural India. *Int J Gynaecol Obstet* **103**:26–29.
Propst AM, Thorp JM Jr (1998) Traumatic vulvar hematomas: conservative versus surgical management. *South Med J* **91**:144–146.

Case 44
Arey ML, Mootha VV, Whittemore AR *et al.* (2007) Computed tomography in the diagnosis of occult open-globe injuries. *Ophthalmology* **114**:1448–1452.

Viestenz A, Schrader W, Küchle M *et al.* (2008) Management of a ruptured globe. *Ophthalmologe* **105**:1163–1174.

Case 45
Scarvelis D, Wells PS (2006) Diagnosis and treatment of deep-vein thrombosis. *Can Med Assoc J* **175**:1087–1092.
Segal JB, Streiff MB, Hofmann LV *et al.* (2007) Management of venous thromboembolism: a systematic review for a practice guideline. *Ann Int Med* **146**:211–222.

Case 46
Kroll MW (2009) Physiology and pathology of TASER electronic control devices. *J Forensic Leg Med* **16**:173–177.
Robb M, Close B, Furyk J *et al.* (2009) Review article: Emergency Department implications of the TASER. *Emerg Med Australas* **21**:250–258.

Case 47
Dogra V, Bhatt S (2004) Acute painful scrotum. *Radiol Clin North Am* **42**:349–363.
Pepe P, Panella P, Pennisi M *et al.* (2006) Does color Doppler sonography improve the clinical assessment of patients with acute scrotum? *Eur J Radiol* **60**:120–124.

Case 48
Hofmeister EP, Kim J, Shin AY (2008) Comparison of 2 methods of immobilization of fifth metacarpal neck fractures: a prospective randomized study. *J Hand Surg* **33**:1362–1368.
Poolman RW, Goslings JC, Lee JB *et al.* (2005) Conservative treatment for closed fifth (small finger) metacarpal neck fractures. *Cochrane Database Syst Rev* **Jul 20**:CD003210.

Further reading

Case 49

Honda H, Warren DK (2009) Central nervous system infections: meningitis and brain abscess. *Infect Dis Clin North Am* **23**:609–623.

van de Beek D (2009) Corticosteroids for acute adult bacterial meningitis. *Méd Maladies Infect* **39**:531–538.

Case 50

Hellinger MD (2002) Anal trauma and foreign bodies. *Surg Clin North Am* **82**:1253–1260.

Ruiz del Castillo J, Sellés Dechent R *et al.* (2001) Colorectal trauma caused by foreign bodies introduced during sexual activity: diagnosis and management. *Rev Esp Enferm Dig* **93**:631–634.

Case 51

Dighe M, Cuevas C, Moshiri M *et al.* (2008) Sonography in first trimester bleeding. *J Clin Ultrasound* **36**:352–366.

Promes SB, Nobay F (2010) Pitfalls in first-trimester bleeding. *Emerg Med Clin North Am* **28**:219–234.

Case 52

Ben Nakhi A, Gupta R, Al-Hunayan A *et al.* (2010) Comparative analysis and interobserver variation of unenhanced computed tomography and intravenous urography in the diagnosis of acute flank pain. *Med Princ Pract* **19**:118–121.

Taourel P, Thuret R, Hoquet M D *et al.* (2008) Computed tomography in the nontraumatic renal causes of acute flank pain. *Semin Ultrasound CT MRI* **29**:341–352.

Case 53

Huang L, Crothers K (2009) HIV-associated opportunistic pneumonias. *Respirology* **14**:474–485.

Krajicek BJ, Thomas CF Jr, Limper AH (2009) Pneumocystis pneumonia: current concepts in pathogenesis, diagnosis, and treatment. *Clin Chest Med* **30**:265–278.

Case 54

Cheong Y, Li TC (2007) Controversies in the management of ectopic pregnancy. *Reprod Biomed Online* **15**:396–402.

Mol F, Mol BW, Ankum WM *et al.* (2008) Current evidence on surgery, systemic methotrexate and expectant management in the treatment of tubal ectopic pregnancy: a systematic review and meta-analysis. *Hum Reprod Update* **14**:309–319.

Case 55

Stein PD, Sostman HD, Bounameaux H *et al.* (2008) Challenges in the diagnosis of acute pulmonary embolism. *Am J Med* **121**:565–571.

Todd JL, Tapson VF (2009) Thrombolytic therapy for acute pulmonary embolism: a critical appraisal. *Chest* **135**:1321–1329.

Case 56

Abul-Kasim K, Selariu E, Brizzi M *et al.* (2009) Hyperdense middle cerebral artery sign in multidetector computed tomography: definition, occurrence, and reliability analysis. *Neurol India* **57**:143–150.

Kharitonova T, Thorén M, Ahmed N *et al.* (2009) Disappearing hyperdense middle cerebral artery sign in ischaemic stroke patients treated with intravenous thrombolysis: clinical course and prognostic significance. *J Neurol Neurosurg Ps* **80**:273–278.

Case 57

McCord J, Jneid H, Hollander JE *et al.* (2008) Management of cocaine-associated chest pain and myocardial infarction: a scientific statement from the American Heart Association Acute Cardiac Care Committee of the Council on Clinical Cardiology. *Circulation* **117**:1897–1907.

Pozner CN, Levine M, Zane R (2005) The cardiovascular effects of cocaine. *J Emerg Med* **29**:173–178.

Case 58

Emery P, McInnes IB, van Vollenhoven R *et al*. (2008) Clinical identification and treatment of a rapidly progressing disease state in patients with rheumatoid arthritis. *Rheumatology* 47:392–398.

Joseph A, Brasington R, Kahl L *et al*. (2010) Immunologic rheumatic disorders. *J Allergy Clin Immunol* 125(Suppl 2):S204–215.

Case 59

Fasanmade OA, Odeniyi IA, Ogbera AO (2008) Diabetic ketoacidosis: diagnosis and management. *Afr J Med Sci* 37:99–105.

Umpierrez GE, Kitabchi AE (2003) Diabetic ketoacidosis: risk factors and management strategies. *Treat Endocrinol* 2:95–108.

Case 60

Anto C, Aradhya P (1996) Clinical diagnosis of peripheral nerve compression in the upper extremity. *Orthop Clin North Am* 27:227–236.

Toussaint CP, Zager EL (2008) What's new in common upper extremity entrapment neuropathies. *Neurosurg Clin North Am* 19:573–581.

Case 61

Blaivas M, Lyon M, Duggal S (2005) A prospective comparison of supine chest radiography and bedside ultrasound for the diagnosis of traumatic pneumothorax. *Acad Emerg Med* 12:844–849.

Soldati G, Testa A, Sher S *et al*. (2008) Occult traumatic pneumothorax: diagnostic accuracy of lung ultrasonography in the emergency department. *Chest* 133:204–211.

Case 62

Cohen PR (2009) Black tongue secondary to bismuth subsalicylate: case report and review of exogenous causes of macular lingual pigmentation. *J Drugs Dermatol* 8:1132–1135.

Ioffreda MD, Gordon CA, Adams DR *et al*. (2001) Black tongue. *Arch Dermatol* 137:968–969.

Case 63

Panda A, Vanathi M, Kumar A *et al*. (2007) Corneal graft rejection. *Surv Ophthalmol* 52:375–396.

Tabbara KF (2008) Pharmacologic strategies in the prevention and treatment of corneal transplant rejection. *Int Ophthalmol* 28:223–232.

Case 64

Garner JP, Meiring PD, Ravi K *et al*. (2007) Psoas abscess – not as rare as we think? *Colorectal Dis* 9:269–274.

Navarro López V, Ramos JM, Meseguer V *et al*. (2009) Microbiology and outcome of iliopsoas abscess in 124 patients. *Medicine* 88:120–130.

Case 65

Narayan S, Thomas CR Jr (2006) Multimodality therapy for Pancoast tumor. *Nat Clin Pract Oncol* 3:484–941.

Rusch VW (2006) Management of Pancoast tumours. *Lancet Oncol* 7:997–1005.

Case 66

Khechinashvili G, Asplund K (2002) Electrocardiographic changes in patients with acute stroke: a systematic review. *Cerebrovasc Dis* 14:67–76.

van Bree MD, Roos YB, van der Bilt IA *et al*. (2010) Prevalence and characterization of ECG abnormalities after intracerebral hemorrhage. *Neurocrit Care* 12:50–55.

Case 67

Belville RG, Seupaul RA (2005) Winged scapula in the emergency department: a case report and review. *J Emerg Med* 29:279–282.

Galano GJ, Bigliani LU, Ahmad CS *et al*. (2008) Surgical treatment of winged scapula. *Clin Orthop Rel Res* 466:652–660.

Further reading

Case 68

Johnson RF, Stewart MG (2005) The contemporary approach to diagnosis and management of peritonsillar abscess. *Curr Opin Otolaryngol Head Neck Surg* **13**:157–160.

Lyon M, Blaivas M (2005) Intraoral ultrasound in the diagnosis and treatment of suspected peritonsillar abscess in the emergency department. *Acad Emerg Med* **12**:85–88.

Case 69

Burns MJ, Linden CH, Graudins A *et al.* (2000) A comparison of physostigmine and benzodiazepines for the treatment of anticholinergic poisoning. *Ann Emerg Med* **35**:374–381.

Göpel C, Laufer C, Marcus A (2002) Three cases of angel's trumpet tea-induced psychosis in adolescent substance abusers. *Nord J Psychiatry* **56**:49–52.

Case 70

Langer MF (2009) Pyogenic flexor tendon sheath infection: a comprehensive review. *Handchir Mikrochir Plast Chir* **41**:256–270.

Small LN, Ross JJ (2005) Suppurative tenosynovitis and septic bursitis. *Infect Dis Clin North Am* **19**:991–1005.

Case 71

Berkowitz RS, Goldstein DP (2009) Clinical practice: molar pregnancy. *New Engl J Med* **360**:1639–1645.

Soper JT (2006) Gestational trophoblastic disease. *Obstet Gynecol* **108**:176–187.

Case 72

Mumcuoglu KY (2001) Clinical applications for maggots in wound care. *Am J Clin Dermatol* **2**:219–227.

Sherman RA, Sherman J, Gilead L *et al.* (2001) Maggot débridement therapy in outpatients. *Arch Phys Med Rehab* **82**:1226–1229.

Case 73

Aerssens J, Paulussen AD (2005) Pharmacogenomics and acquired long QT syndrome. *Pharmacogenomics* **6**:259–270.

Chiang CE (2004) Congenital and acquired long QT syndrome: current concepts and management. *Cardiol Rev* **12**:222–234.

Case 74

Nguyen DH, Martin JT (2008) Common dental infections in the primary care setting. *Am Fam Physician* **77**:797–802.

Wayne DB, Trajtenberg CP, Hyman DJ (2001) Tooth and periodontal disease: a review for the primary-care physician. *South Med J* **94**:925–932.

Case 75

Benson DW (2004) Genetics of atrioventricular conduction disease in humans. *Anat Rec A Discov Mol Cell Evol Biol* **280**:934–939.

Lee S, Wellens HJ, Josephson ME (2009) Paroxysmal atrioventricular block. *Heart Rhythm* **6**:1229–1234.

Case 76

Schlesinger N (2005) Diagnosis of gout: clinical, laboratory, and radiologic findings. *Am J Manag Care* **11(15 Suppl)**:S443–450.

Schlesinger N (2007) Diagnosis of gout. *Minerva Med* **98**:759–767.

Case 77

Groh GI, Wirth MA, Rockwood CA Jr (2010) Results of treatment of luxatio erecta (inferior shoulder dislocation). *J Shoulder Elbow Surg* **19**:423–426.

Nho SJ, Dodson CC, Bardzik KF *et al.* (2006) The two-step maneuver for closed reduction of inferior glenohumeral dislocation (luxatio erecta to anterior dislocation to reduction). *J Ortho Trauma* **20**:354–357.

Case 78

Brooks A, Davies B, Smethhurst M *et al.* (2004) Emergency ultrasound in the acute assessment of haemothorax. *Emerg Med J* **21**:44–46.

Rippey JC, Royse AG (2009) Ultrasound in trauma. *Best Pract Res Clin Anaesthesiol* **23**:343–362.

Case 79

Myers KA, Farquhar DR (2001) The rational clinical examination. Does this patient have clubbing? *J Am Med Assoc* **286**:341–347.

Spicknall KE, Zirwas MJ, English JC 3rd (2005) Clubbing: an update on diagnosis, differential diagnosis, pathophysiology, and clinical relevance. *J Am Acad Dermatol* **52**:1020–1028.

Case 80

Stell IM (1996) Septic and non-septic olecranon bursitis in the accident and emergency department: an approach to management. *J Accid Emerg Med* **13**:351–353.

Stell IM (1999) Management of acute bursitis: outcome study of a structured approach. *J R Soc Med* **92**:516–521.

Case 81

Bastos R, Baisden CE, Harker L *et al.* (2008) Penetrating thoracic trauma. *Sem Thorac Cardiovasc Surg* **20**:19–25.

Keel M, Meier C (2007) Chest injuries: what is new? *Curr Opin Crit Care* **13**:674–679.

Case 82

Gilchrist JM (2009) Seventh cranial neuropathy. *Sem Neurol* **29**:5–13.

Sweeney CJ, Gilden DH (2001) Ramsay Hunt syndrome. *J Neurol Neurosurg Psychiatry* **71**:149–154.

Case 83

Saber AA, Boros MJ (2005) Chilaiditi's syndrome: what should every surgeon know? *Am Surg* **71**:261–263.

Sato M, Ishida H, Konno K *et al.* (2000) Chilaiditi syndrome: sonographic findings. *Abdom Imaging* **25**:397–399.

Case 84

Arikan S, Kocakusak A, Yucel AF *et al.* (2005) A prospective comparison of the selective observation and routine exploration methods for penetrating abdominal stab wounds with organ or omentum evisceration. *J Trauma* **58**:526–532.

da Silva M, Navsaria PH, Edu S *et al.* (2009) Evisceration following abdominal stab wounds: analysis of 66 cases. *World J Surg* **33**:215–219.

Case 85

Geissler WB (2005) Intra-articular distal radius fractures: the role of arthroscopy? *Hand Clin* **21**:407–416.

Ng CY, McQueen MM (2011) What are the radiological predictors of functional outcome following fractures of the distal radius? *J Bone Joint Surg Br* **93**:145–150.

Case 86

Ashe MC, McCauley T, Khan KM (2004) Tendinopathies in the upper extremity: a paradigm shift. *J Hand Ther* **17**:329–334.

Richie CA 3rd, Briner WW Jr (2003) Corticosteroid injection for treatment of de Quervain's tenosynovitis: a pooled quantitative literature evaluation. *J Am Board Fam Pract* **16**:102–106.

Case 87

Sicherer SH, Leung DY (2009) Advances in allergic skin disease, anaphylaxis, and hypersensitivity reactions to foods, drugs, and insects in 2008. *J Allergy Clin Immunol* **123**:319–327.

Simons FE (2009) Anaphylaxis: recent advances in assessment and treatment. *J Allergy Clin Immunol* **124**:625–636.

Further reading

Case 88

Jenny JY, Boeri C, El Amrani H *et al.* (2005) Should plain X-rays be routinely performed after blunt knee trauma? A prospective analysis. *J Trauma* **58**:1179–1182.

Robb G, Reid D, Arroll B *et al.* (2007) General practitioner diagnosis and management of acute knee injuries: summary of an evidence-based guideline. *New Z Med J* **120(1249)**:U2419.

Case 89

Li XF, Dai LY, Lu H *et al.* (2006) A systematic review of the management of hangman's fractures. *Eur Spine J* **15**:257–269.

Pratt H, Davies E, King L (2008) Traumatic injuries of the c1/c2 complex: computed tomographic imaging appearances. *Curr Prob Diag Radiol* **37**:26–38.

Case 90

Brusin JH (2008) Osteogenesis imperfecta. *Radiol Tech* **79**:535–548.

Phillipi CA, Remmington T, Steiner RD (2008) Bisphosphonate therapy for osteogenesis imperfecta. *Cochrane Database Syst Rev* **8**:CD005088.

Case 91

Jiamsripong P, Mookadam F, Oh JK *et al.* (2009) Spectrum of pericardial disease: part II. *Expert Rev Cardiovasc Ther* **7**:1159–1169.

Mookadam F, Jiamsripong P, Oh JK *et al.* (2009) Spectrum of pericardial disease: part I. *Expert Rev Cardiovasc Ther* **7**:1149–1157.

Case 92

Diamantopoulos II, Jones NS (2001) The investigation of nasal septal perforations and ulcers. *J Laryngol Otol* **115**:541–544.

Lanier B, Kai G, Marple B *et al.* (2007) Pathophysiology and progression of nasal septal perforation. *Ann Allergy Asthma Immunol* **99**:473–4.

Case 93

Gerding DN, Muto CA, Owens RC Jr (2008) Treatment of *Clostridium difficile* infection. *Clin Infect Dis* **46(Suppl 1)**:S32–42.

Kelly CP (2009) A 76-year-old man with recurrent *Clostridium difficile*-associated diarrhea: review of *C. difficile* infection. *J Am Med Assoc* **301**:954–962.

Case 94

Laborderie J, Barandon L, Ploux S *et al.* (2008) Management of subacute and delayed right ventricular perforation with a pacing or an implantable cardioverter-defibrillator lead. *Am J Cardiol* **102**:1352–1355.

Sterliński M, Przybylski A, Maciag A *et al.* (2009) Subacute cardiac perforations associated with active fixation leads. *Europace* **11**:206–212.

Case 95

Durkin A, Sagi HC, Durham R *et al.* (2006) Contemporary management of pelvic fractures. *Am J Surg* **192**:211–223.

Metz CM, Hak DJ, Goulet JA *et al.* (2004) Pelvic fracture patterns and their corresponding angiographic sources of hemorrhage. *Orthop Clin North Am* **35**:431–437.

Case 96

Marx JJ, Thömke F (2009) Classical crossed brain stem syndromes: myth or reality? *J Neurol* **256**:898–903.

Norrving B, Hydén D (2004) New aspects of Wallenberg syndrome and other brain stem infarctions. *Lakartidningen* **101**:2728–2730, 2732, 2734.

Case 97

Evans BG, Evans GR (2008) MOC-PSSM CME article: zygomatic fractures. *Plast Reconstr Surg* **121(1 Suppl)**:1–11.

Schubert W, Jenabzadeh K (2009) Endoscopic approach to maxillofacial trauma. *J Craniofac Surgery* **20**:154–156.

Case 98

Gosens T, Hofstee DJ (2009) Calcifying tendinitis of the shoulder: advances in imaging and management. *Curr Rheumatol Rep* **11**:129–134.

Hurt G, Baker CL Jr (2003) Calcific tendinitis of the shoulder. *Orthop Clin North Am* **34**:567–575.

Case 99

Canzanello VJ, Hylander-Rossner B, Sands RE *et al.* (1991) Comparison of 50% dextrose water, 25% mannitol, and 23.5% saline for the treatment of hemodialysis-associated muscle cramps. *Tr Am Soc Artif Intern Organ* **37**:649–652.

Sherman RA, Goodling KA, Eisinger RP (1982) Acute therapy of hemodialysis-related muscle cramps. *Am J Kidney Dis* **2**:287–288.

Case 100

Attasaranya S, Fogel EL, Lehman GA (2008) Choledocholithiasis, ascending cholangitis, and gallstone pancreatitis. *Med Clin North Am* **92**:925–960.

van Erpecum KJ (2006) Gallstone disease: complications of bile-duct stones: acute cholangitis and pancreatitis. *Best Pract Res Clin Gastroenterol* **20**:1139–1152.

Case 101

Benson LS, Edwards SL, Schiff A P *et al.* (2006) Dog and cat bites to the hand: treatment and cost assessment. *J Hand Surg* **31**:468–473.

Dendle C, Looke D (2009) Management of mammalian bites. *Aust Fam Physician* **38**:868–874.

Case 102

Khan S, Kundi A, Sharieff S (2004) Prevalence of right ventricular myocardial infarction in patients with acute inferior wall myocardial infarction. *Int J Clin Pract* **58**:354–357.

Kukla P, Dudek D, Rakowski T *et al.* (2006) Inferior wall myocardial infarction with or without right ventricular involvement: treatment and in-hospital course. *Kardiol Pol* **64**:583–588.

Case 103

Garner JP, Jenner J, Parkhouse DA (2005) Prediction of upper airway closure in inhalational injury. *Mil Med* **170**:677–682.

Leon-Villapalos J, Jeschke MG, Herndon DN (2008) Topical management of facial burns. *Burns* **34**:903–911.

Case 104

Esmeili T, Lozada-Nur F, Epstein J (2005) Common benign oral soft tissue masses. *Dent Clin North Am* **49**:223–240.

Stoopler ET, Sollecito TP, Greenberg MS (2003) Seizure disorders: update of medical and dental considerations. *Gen Dent* **51**:361–366

Case 105

Bouillon R (2006) Acute adrenal insufficiency. *Endocrinol Metab Clin North Am* **35**:767–775.

Hahner S, Allolio B (2005) Management of adrenal insufficiency in different clinical settings. *Expert Opin Pharmacother* **6**:2407–2417.

Case 106

Coche E, Verschuren F, Hainaut P *et al.* (2004) Pulmonary embolism findings on chest radiographs and multislice spiral CT. *Eur Radiol* **14**:1241–1248.

Stein PD, Afzal A, Henry J W *et al.* (2000) Fever in acute pulmonary embolism. *Chest* **117**:39–42.

Case 107

Armstrong TS, Gilbert MR (2000) Metastatic brain tumors: diagnosis, treatment, and nursing interventions. *Clin J Oncol Nurs* **4**:217–225.

Further reading

Buckner JC, Brown PD, O'Neill BP *et al.* (2007) Central nervous system tumors. *Mayo Clin Proc* **82**:1271–1286.

Case 108

Holmes DR Jr, Nishimura R, Fountain R *et al.* (2009) Iatrogenic pericardial effusion and tamponade in the percutaneous intracardiac intervention era. *J Am Coll Cardiol: Cardiovasc Interv* **2**:705–717.

Seferovi PM, Risti AD, Imazio M *et al.* (2006) Management strategies in pericardial emergencies. *Herz* **31**:891–900.

Case 109

Reddy VG (2005) Auto-PEEP: how to detect and how to prevent: a review. *Middle East J Anesthesiol* **18**:293–312.

Segal E (2007) Intrinsic positive end expiratory pressure (PEEP) in mechanically ventilated patients. *Harefuah* **146**:790–793, 812–813.

Case 110

Edlich RF, Winters KL, Britt LD *et al.* (2005) Bacterial diseases of the skin. *J Long-Term Eff Med Implants* **15**:499–510.

Trent JT, Federman D, Kirsner RS (2001) Common bacterial skin infections. *Ostomy Wound Manage* **47**:30–34.

Case 111

Holstein A, Beil W (2009) Oral antidiabetic drug metabolism: pharmacogenomics and drug interactions. *Expert Opin Drug Metab Toxicol* **5**:225–241.

Murad MH, Coto-Yglesias F, Wang AT *et al.* (2009) Clinical review: drug-induced hypoglycemia: a systematic review. *J Clin Endocrinol Metab* **94**:741–745.

Case 112

Aronow WS (2008) Etiology, pathophysiology, and treatment of atrial fibrillation: part 1. *Cardiol Rev* **16**:181–188.

Khoo CW, Lip GY (2009) Acute management of atrial fibrillation. *Chest* **135**:849–859.

Case 113

Ebright JR, Pieper B (2002) Skin and soft tissue infections in injection drug users. *Infect Dis Clin North Am* **16**:697–712.

Korownyk C, Allan GM (2007) Evidence-based approach to abscess management. *Can Fam Physician* **53**:1680–1684.

Case 114

Sgarbossa EB, Pinski SL, Barbagelata A *et al.* (1996) Electrocardiographic diagnosis of evolving acute myocardial infarction in the presence of left bundle-branch block: GUSTO-1 (Global Utilization of Streptokinase and Tissue Plasminogen Activator for Occluded Coronary Arteries) Investigators. *N Engl J Med* **334**:481–487.

Tabas JA, Rodriguez RM, Seligman HK *et al.* (2008) Electrocardiographic criteria for detecting acute myocardial infarction in patients with left bundle branch block: a meta-analysis. *Ann Emerg Med* **52**:329–336.

Case 115

Lal SK, Morgenstern R, Vinjirayer EP *et al.* (2006) Sigmoid volvulus an update. *Gastrointest Endoscopy Clin North Am* **16**:175–187.

Safioleas M, Chatziconstantinou C, Felekouras E *et al.* (2007) Clinical considerations and therapeutic strategy for sigmoid volvulus in the elderly: a study of 33 cases. *World J Gastroenterol* **13**:921–924.

Case 116

Grodski S, Serpell J (2008) Evidence for the role of perioperative PTH measurement after total thyroidectomy as a predictor of hypocalcemia. *World J Surg* **32**:1367–1373.

Testini M, Gurrado A, Lissidini G *et al.* (2007) Hypoparathyroidism after total thyroidectomy. *Minerva Chir* 62:409–415.

Case 117
Coons MS, Green SM (1995) Boutonniere deformity. *Hand Clin* 11:387–402.
Towfigh H, Gruber P (2005) Surgical treatment of the boutonnière deformity. *Oper Orthop Traumatol* 17:66–78.

Case 118
Dighe M, Cuevas C, Moshiri M *et al.* (2008) Sonography in first trimester bleeding. *J Clin Ultrasound* 36:352–366.
Dogra V, Paspulati RM, Bhatt S (2005) First trimester bleeding evaluation. *Ultrasound Q* 21:69–85.

Case 119
Bardin T (2003) Gonococcal arthritis. *Best Pract Res Clin Rheumatol* 17:201–208.
Rice PA (2005) Gonococcal arthritis (disseminated gonococcal infection). *Infect Dis Clin North Am* 19:853–861.

Case 120
Ariyarajah V, Jassal DS, Kirkpatrick I *et al.* (2009) The utility of cardiovascular magnetic resonance in constrictive pericardial disease. *Cardiol Rev* 17:77–82.
Schwefer M, Aschenbach R, Heidemann J *et al.* (2009) Constrictive pericarditis, still a diagnostic challenge: comprehensive review of clinical management. *Eur J Cardiothorac Surg* 36:502–510.

Case 121
Kovalyshyn I, Busam KJ, Marghoob AA (2009) Orange-yellow diffuse cutaneous eruption in an 82-year-old woman. *Arch Dermatol* 145:1183–1188.
Lugo-Somolinos A, Sánchez JE (2003) Xanthomas: a marker for hyperlipidemias. *Bol Asoc Med P R* 95:12–16.

Case 122
Krajewski W, Kucharska M, Pilacik B *et al.* (2007) Impaired vitamin B12 metabolic status in healthcare workers occupationally exposed to nitrous oxide. *Br J Anaesth* 99:812–818.
Weimann J (2003) Toxicity of nitrous oxide. *Best Pract Res Clin Anaesthesiol* 17:47–61.

Case 123
Focht A, Jones AE, Lowe TJ (2009) Early goal-directed therapy: improving mortality and morbidity of sepsis in the emergency department. *Jt Comm J Qual Patient Saf* 35:186–191.
Wheeler AP (2007) Recent developments in the diagnosis and management of severe sepsis. *Chest* 132:1967–1976.

Case 124
Bellapianta JM, Ljungquist K, Tobin E *et al.* (2009) Necrotizing fasciitis. *J Am Acad Orthop Surg* 17:174–182.
Sarani B, Strong M, Pascual J *et al.* (2009) Necrotizing fasciitis: current concepts and review of the literature. *J Am Coll Surg* 208:279–288.

Case 125
Capaccio P, Torretta S, Ottavian F *et al.* (2007) Modern management of obstructive salivary diseases. *Acta Otorhinolaryngol Ital* 27:161–172.
McGurk M, Escudier MP, Brown E (2004) Modern management of obstructive salivary gland disease. *Ann R Australas Coll Dent Surg* 17:45–50.

Case 126
Nord RM, Quach T, Walsh M *et al.* (2009) Detection of traumatic arthrotomy of the knee using the saline solution load test. *J Bone Joint Surg Am Vol* 91:66–70.
Tornetta P 3rd, Boes MT, Schepsis AA *et al.* (2008) How effective is a saline arthrogram for wounds around the knee? *Clin Orthop Rel Res* 466:432–435.

Further reading

Case 127

Hoare C, Li Wan Po A, Williams H (2000) Systematic review of treatments for atopic eczema. *Health Technol Assess* 4:1–191.

Roos TC, Geuer S, Roos S *et al.* (2004) Recent advances in treatment strategies for atopic dermatitis. *Drugs* 64:2639–2666.

Case 128

Benson DW (2004) Genetics of atrioventricular conduction disease in humans. *Anat Rec A Discov Mol Cell Evol Biol* 280:934–939.

Drew BJ (2006) Pitfalls and artifacts in electrocardiography. *Cardiol Clin* 24:309–315.

Case 129

Bord SP, Linden J (2008) Trauma to the globe and orbit. *Emerg Med Clin North Am* 26:97–123.

Kontio R, Lindqvist C (2009) Management of orbital fractures. *Oral Maxillofac Surg Clin North Am* 21:209–220.

Case 130

Bar-Natan M, Salai M, Sidi Y *et al.* (2002) Sternoclavicular infectious arthritis in previously healthy adults. *Semin Arthritis Rheum* 32:189–195.

Ross JJ, Shamsuddin H (2004) Sternoclavicular septic arthritis: review of 180 cases. *Medicine* 83:139–148.

Case 131

De Luca L, Fonarow GC, Adams KF Jr *et al.* (2007) Acute heart failure syndromes: clinical scenarios and pathophysiologic targets for therapy. *Heart Fail Rev* 12:97–104.

Gheorghiade M, Pang PS (2009) Acute heart failure syndromes. *J Am Coll Cardiol* 53:557–573.

Case 132

Anon (2005) Chickenpox vaccines: new drugs. A favourable risk-benefit balance in some situations. *Prescrire Int* 14:85–91.

Tunbridge AJ, Breuer J, Jeffery KJ (2008) Chickenpox in adults: clinical management. *J Infect* 57:95–102.

Case 133

Davila ML (2006) Neutropenic enterocolitis. *Curr Opin Gastroenterol* 22:44–47.

Ullery BW, Pieracci FM, Rodney JR *et al.* (2009) Neutropenic enterocolitis. *Surg Infect* 10:307–314.

Case 134

Lavonas EJ, Schaeffer TH, Kokko J *et al.* (2009) Crotaline Fab antivenom appears to be effective in cases of severe North American pit viper envenomation: an integrative review. *BMC Emerg Med* 9:13.

Singletary EM, Rochman AS, Bodmer JC *et al.* (2005) Envenomations. *Med Clin North Am* 89:1195–1224.

Case 135

Kerns W 2nd (2007) Management of beta-adrenergic blocker and calcium channel antagonist toxicity. *Emerg Med Clin North Am* 25:309–331.

Shepherd G (2006) Treatment of poisoning caused by beta-adrenergic and calcium-channel blockers. *Am J Health Syst Pharm* 63:1828–1835.

Case 136

Coetzee JC (2008) Making sense of lisfranc injuries. *Foot Ankle Clin* 13:695–704.

DeOrio M, Erickson M, Usuelli FG *et al.* (2009) Lisfranc injuries in sport. *Foot Ankle Clin* 14:169–186.

Case 137

Brilliant LC, Grillo A (1993) Successful resuscitation from cardiopulmonary arrest following deliberate inhalation of Freon refrigerant gas. *Del Med J* 65:375–378.

Sabik LM, Abbas RA, Ismail MM *et al.* (2009) Cardiotoxicity of freon among refrigeration services workers: comparative cross-sectional study. *Environ Health* 8:31.

Case 138

Kregor PJ, Templeman D (2002) Associated injuries complicating the management of acetabular fractures: review and case studies. *Orthop Clin North Am* 33:73–95.

Yang EC, Cornwall R (2000) Initial treatment of traumatic hip dislocations in the adult. *Clin Orthop Rel Res* 377:24–31.

Case 139

Marderstein EL, Delaney CP (2007) Surgical management of rectal prolapse. *Nat Clin Pract Gastroenterol Hepatol* 4:552–561.

Purkayastha S, Tekkis P, Athanasiou T *et al.* (2005) A comparison of open vs laparoscopic abdominal rectopexy for full-thickness rectal prolapse: a meta-analysis. *Dis Colon Rectum* 48:1930–1940.

Case 140

Cherington M, McDonough G, Olson S *et al.* (2007) Lichtenberg figures and lightning: case reports and review of the literature. *Cutis* 80:141–143.

Ritenour AE, Morton MJ, McManus JG *et al.* (2008) Lightning injury: a review. *Burns* 34:585–594.

Case 141

El-Hemaidi I, Gharaibeh A, Shehata H (2007) Menorrhagia and bleeding disorders. *Curr Opin Obstetr Gynecol* 19:513–520.

Kadir RA, Chi C (2006) Women and von Willebrand disease: controversies in diagnosis and management. *Semin Thromb Hemost* 32:605–615.

Case 142

Bullock MR, Chesnut R, Ghajar J *et al.* (2006) Surgical management of acute subdural hematomas. *Neurosurgery* 58(3 Suppl):S16–24.

Valadka AB, Robertson CS (2007) Surgery of cerebral trauma and associated critical care. *Neurosurgery* 61(1 Suppl):203–220.

Case 143

Langell JT, Mulvihill SJ (2008) Gastrointestinal perforation and the acute abdomen. *Med Clin North Am* 92:599–625.

Lüning TH, Keemers-Gels ME, Barendregt WB *et al.* (2007) Colonoscopic perforations: a review of 30,366 patients. *Surg Endosc* 21:994–997.

Case 144

Charytan D, Jansen K (2003) Severe metabolic complications from theophylline intoxication. *Nephrology* 8:239–242.

McCord J, Borzak S (1998) Multifocal atrial tachycardia. *Chest* 113:203–209.

Case 145

Hazin R, Ibrahimi OA, Hazin MI *et al.* (2008) Stevens-Johnson syndrome: pathogenesis, diagnosis, and management. *Ann Med* 40:129–138.

Lamoreux MR, Sternbach MR, Hsu WT (2006) Erythema multiforme. *Am Fam Physician* 74:1883–1888.

Case 146

Golant A, Nord RM, Paksima N *et al.* (2008) Cold exposure injuries to the extremities. *J Am Acad Orthop Surg* 16:704–715.

Long WB 3rd, Edlich RF, Winters KL *et al.* (2005) Cold injuries. *J Long-Term Eff Med Implants* 15:67–78.

Further reading

Case 147
Baikoussis NG, Apostolakis EE (2010)
Penetrating atherosclerotic ulcer of the
thoracic aorta: diagnosis and treatment.
Hellenic J Cardiol **51**:153–157.
de Souza DG, Blank RS, Mazzeo FJ *et al.*
(2009) Penetrating ascending aortic
atherosclerotic ulcer. *Anesth Analg*
109:1035–1037.

Case 148
Carley SD (2003) Beyond the 12 lead:
review of the use of additional leads for
the early electrocardiographic diagnosis
of acute myocardial infarction. *Emerg
Med* **15**:143–154.
Menon V, Harrington RA, Hochman JS *et
al.* (2004) Thrombolysis and adjunctive
therapy in acute myocardial infarction:
the Seventh ACCP Conference on
Antithrombotic and Thrombolytic
Therapy. *Chest* **126(3 Suppl)**:549S–575S.

Case 149
Tuli SS, Schultz GS, Downer DM (2007)
Science and strategy for preventing and
managing corneal ulceration. *Ocul Surf*
5:23–39.
Wirbelauer C (2006) Management of the
red eye for the primary care physician.
Am J Med **119**:302–306.

Case 150
Kashefi C, Messer K, Barden R *et al.*
(2008) Incidence and prevention of
iatrogenic urethral injuries. *J Urol*
179:2254–2257.
Maheshwari PN, Shah HN (2005)
Immediate endoscopic management of
complete iatrogenic anterior urethral
injuries: a case series with long-term
results. *BMC Urol* **5**:13.

Case 151
Freitas ML, Bell RL, Duffy AJ (2006)
Choledocholithiasis: evolving standards
for diagnosis and management. *World J
Gastroenterol* **12**:3162–3167.

Martin DJ, Vernon DR, Toouli J (2006)
Surgical versus endoscopic treatment of
bile duct stones. *Cochrane Database Syst
Rev* **Apr 19;(2)**:CD003327.

Case 152
Hankins DG, Rosekrans JA (2004)
Overview, prevention, and treatment of
rabies. *Mayo Clin Proc* **79**:671–676.
Warrell MJ, Warrell DA (2004) Rabies and
other lyssavirus diseases. *Lancet*
363:959–969.

Case 153
Tanous D, Benson LN, Horlick EM (2009)
Coarctation of the aorta: evaluation and
management. *Curr Opin Cardiol*
24:509–515.
Vohra HA, Adamson L, Haw MP (2009)
Does surgical correction of coarctation of
the aorta in adults reduce established
hypertension? *Interact Cardiovasc
Thorac Surg* **8**:123–127.

Case 154
Egol K, Walsh M, Rosenblatt K *et al.*
(2007) Avulsion fractures of the fifth
metatarsal base: a prospective outcome
study. *Foot Ankle Int* **28**:581–583.
Rammelt S, Heineck J, Zwipp H (2004)
Metatarsal fractures. *Injury*
35(Suppl 2):SB77–86.

Case 155
Cannon J, Silvestri S, Munro M (2009)
Imaging choices in occult hip fracture. *J
Emerg Med* **37**:144–152.
Perron AD, Miller MD, Brady WJ (2002)
Orthopedic pitfalls in the ED:
radiographically occult hip fracture. *Am
J Emerg Med* **20**:234–237.

Case 156
Byrd JB, Adam A, Brown NJ (2006)
Angiotensin-converting enzyme inhibitor-
associated angioedema. *Immunol Allergy
Clin North Am* **26**:725–737.

Malde B, Regalado J, Greenberger PA (2007) Investigation of angioedema associated with the use of angiotensin-converting enzyme inhibitors and angiotensin receptor blockers. *Ann Allergy Asthma Immunol* 98:57–63.

Case 157

Karnath BM, Champion JC, Ahmad M (2003) Electrocardiographic manifestations of proximal left anterior descending artery occlusion. *J Electrocardiol* 36:173–177.

Rhinehardt J, Brady WJ, Perron AD *et al.* (2002) Electrocardiographic manifestations of Wellens' syndrome. *Am J Emerg Med* 20:638–643.

Case 158

Frink M, Hildebrand F, Krettek C *et al.* (2010) Compartment syndrome of the lower leg and foot. *Clin Orthop Rel Res* 468:940–950.

Shadgan B, Menon M, O'Brien PJ *et al.* (2008) Diagnostic techniques in acute compartment syndrome of the leg. *J Orthop Trauma* 22:581–587.

Case 159

Batke M, Cappell MS (2008) Adynamic ileus and acute colonic pseudo-obstruction. *Med Clin North Am* 92:649–670.

Cappell MS, Batke M (2008) Mechanical obstruction of the small bowel and colon. *Med Clin North Am* 92:575–597.

Case 160

Campochiaro PA (2004) Ocular neovascularisation and excessive vascular permeability. *Expert Opin Biol Ther* 4:1395–1402.

Safvati A, Cole N, Hume E *et al.* (2009) Mediators of neovascularization and the hypoxic cornea. *Curr Eye Res* 34:501–514.

Case 161

Graeber B, Vanderwal T, Stiller R *et al.* (2005) Late postpartum eclampsia as an obstetric complication seen in the ED. *Am J Emerg Med* 23:168–170.

Karumanchi SA, Lindheimer MD (2008) Advances in the understanding of eclampsia. *Curr Hypertens Rep* 10:305–312.

Case 162

Giblin AV, Clover AJ, Athanassopoulos A *et al.* (2007) Pyogenic granuloma: the quest for optimum treatment: audit of treatment of 408 cases. *J Plast Reconstr Aesthet Surg* 60:1030–1035.

Lin RL, Janniger CK (2004) Pyogenic granuloma. *Cutis* 74:229–233.

Case 163

Koplan BA, Stevenson WG (2009) Ventricular tachycardia and sudden cardiac death. *Mayo Clin Proc* 84:289–297.

Srivathsan K, Ng DW, Mookadam F (2009) Ventricular tachycardia and ventricular fibrillation. *Exp Rev Cardiovasc Ther* 7:801–809.

Case 164

Barakat M, Belkhadir ZH, Belkrezia R *et al.* (2004) Traumatic asphyxia or Perthe's syndrome: six case reports. *Ann Fr Anesth Reanim* 23:59–62.

Esme H, Solak O, Yurumez Y *et al.* (2006) Perthes syndrome associated with bilateral optic disc edema. *Can J Ophthalmol* 41:780–782.

Case 165

Holdgate A, Foo A (2006) Adenosine versus intravenous calcium channel antagonists for the treatment of supraventricular tachycardia in adults. *Cochrane Database Syst Rev* 18:CD005154.

Further reading

McGuire MA (2007) Paroxysmal supraventricular tachycardia: a century of progress. *Heart Lung Circ* **16**:222–228.

Case 166

Al-Shahi R, Warlow C (2001) A systematic review of the frequency and prognosis of arteriovenous malformations of the brain in adults. *Brain* **124**:1900–1926.

Al-Shahi R, Warlow CP (2006) Interventions for treating brain arteriovenous malformations in adults. *Cochrane Database Syst Rev* **25**:CD003436.

Case 167

Arslan U, Balcio lu S, Tavil Y *et al.* (2008) Clinical and angiographic importance of right bundle branch block in the setting of acute anterior myocardial infarction. *Anatol J Cardiol* **8**:123–127.

Kurisu S, Inoue I, Kawagoe T *et al.* (2007) Right bundle-branch block in anterior acute myocardial infarction in the coronary intervention era: acute angiographic findings and prognosis. *Int J Cardiol* **116**:57–61.

Case 168

Moawad NS, Mahajan ST, Moniz MH *et al.* (2010) Current diagnosis and treatment of interstitial pregnancy. *Am J Obstet Gynecol* **202**:15–29.

Ross R, Lindheim SR, Olive DL *et al.* (2006) Cornual gestation: a systematic literature review and two case reports of a novel treatment regimen. *J Minim Invasive Gynecol* **13**:74–78.

Case 169

Franchini M (2006) Thrombotic microangiopathies: an update. *Hematology* **11**:139–146.

Patel A, Patel H, Patel A (2009) Thrombotic thrombocytopenic purpura: the masquerader. *South Med J* **102**:504–509.

Case 170

Campos GM, Vittinghoff E, Rabl C *et al.* (2009) Endoscopic and surgical treatments for achalasia: a systematic review and meta-analysis. *Ann Surg* **249**:45–57.

Wang L, Li YM, Li L (2009) Meta-analysis of randomized and controlled treatment trials for achalasia. *Dig Dis Sci* **54**:2303–2311.

Case 171

Kasten P, Schewe B, Maurer F *et al.* (2001) Rupture of the patellar tendon: a review of 68 cases and a retrospective study of 29 ruptures comparing two methods of augmentation. *Arch Orthop Trauma Surg* **121**:578–582.

Ramseier LE, Werner CM, Heinzelmann M (2006) Quadriceps and patellar tendon rupture. *Injury* **37**:516–519.

Case 172

Eren S, Kantarci M, Okur A (2006) Imaging of diaphragmatic rupture after trauma. *Clin Radiol* **61**:467–477.

Scharff JR, Naunheim KS (2007) Traumatic diaphragmatic injuries. *Thorac Surg Clin* **17**:81–85.

Case 173

Brown MA (2008) Imaging acute appendicitis. *Semin Ultrasound CT MI* **29**:293–307.

Rybkin AV, Thoeni RF (2007) Current concepts in imaging of appendicitis. *Radiol Clin North Am* **45**:411–422.

Case 174

Horne BR, Corley FG (2008) Review of 88 nail gun injuries to the extremities. *Injury* **39**:357–361.

Hussey K, Knox D, Lambah A *et al.* (2008) Nail gun injuries to the hand. *J Trauma* **64**:170–173.

Case 175

Elston DM (2007) Aquatic antagonists: Portuguese man-of-war (*Physalia physalis*). *Cutis* **80**:186–188.

Loten C, Stokes B, Worsley D *et al.* (2006) A randomised controlled trial of hot water (45 degrees C) immersion versus ice packs for pain relief in bluebottle stings. *Med J Aust* **184:**329–333.

Case 176
Muñoz FJ, Mismetti P, Poggio R *et al.* (2008) Clinical outcome of patients with upper-extremity deep vein thrombosis: results from the RIETE Registry. *Chest* **133:**143–148.
Sajid MS, Ahmed N, Desai M *et al.* (2007) Upper limb deep vein thrombosis: a literature review to streamline the protocol for management. *Acta Haematol* **118:**10–18.

Case 177
Bonnetblanc JM, Bédane C (2003) Erysipelas: recognition and management. *Am J Clin Dermatol* **4:**157–163.
Gabillot-Carré M, Roujeau JC (2007) Acute bacterial skin infections and cellulitis. *Curr Opin Infect Dis* **20:**118–123.

Case 178
Kindermann M, Schwaab B, Berg M *et al.* (2001) Longevity of dual chamber pacemakers: device and patient related determinants. *Pacing Clin Electrophysiol* **24:**810–815.
Ribeiro AL, Rincón LG, Oliveira BG *et al.* (2001) Enhancing longevity of pacemakers through reprogramming: underutilization and cost-effectiveness. *Arq Bras Cardiol* **76:**437–444.

Case 179
Byrd JA, Bruce AJ, Rogers RS 3rd (2003) Glossitis and other tongue disorders. *Dermatol Clin* **21:**123–134.
Gonsalves WC, Chi AC, Neville BW (2007) Common oral lesions: Part I: superficial mucosal lesions. *Am Fam Physician* **75:**501–507.

Case 180
Deininger MH, Adam A, Van Velthoven V (2008) Free-hand bedside catheter evacuation of cerebellar hemorrhage. *Minim Invasive Neurosurg* **51:**57–60.
Jensen MB, St Louis EK (2005) Management of acute cerebellar stroke. *Arch Neurol* **62:**537–544.

Case 181
Dourmishev LA, Dourmishev AL (2005) Syphilis: uncommon presentations in adults. *Clin Dermatol* **23:**555–564.
Lautenschlager S (2006) Cutaneous manifestations of syphilis: recognition and management. *Am J Clin Dermatol* **7:**291–304.

Case 182
Ladner HE, Danielsen B, Gilbert WM (2005) Acute myocardial infarction in pregnancy and the puerperium: a population-based study. *Obstet Gynecol* **105:**480–484.
Lodha A, Mirsakov N, Malik B *et al.* (2009) Spontaneous coronary artery dissection: case report and review of literature. *South Med J* **102:**315–317.

Case 183
Mahboob A, Haroon TS (1998) Drugs causing fixed eruptions: a study of 450 cases. *Int J Dermatol* **37:**833–838.
Ozkaya E (2008) Fixed drug eruption: state of the art. *J Dtsch Dermatol Ges* **6:**181–188.

Case 184
Kirchoff C, Stegmaier J, Volkering C *et al.* (2007) Diagnosis and treatment of paronychia. *MMW Fortschr Med* **149:**34–35.
Rigopoulos D, Larios G, Gregoriou S *et al.* (2008) Acute and chronic paronychia. *Am Fam Physician* **77:**339–346.

Further reading

Case 185

Antonio-Santos AA, Santo RN *et al.* (2005) Pharmacological testing of anisocoria. *Expert Opin Pharmacother* 6:2007–2013.

Moeller JJ, Maxner CE (2007) The dilated pupil: an update. *Curr Neurol Neurosci Rep* 7:417–422.

Case 186

Haan JM, Bochicchio GV, Kramer N *et al.* (2005) Nonoperative management of blunt splenic injury: a 5-year experience. *J Trauma* 58:492–498.

Harbrecht BG (2005) Is anything new in adult blunt splenic trauma? *Am J Surg* 190:273–278.

Case 187

Lin CC, Chen KF, Shih CP *et al.* (2008) The prognostic factors of hypotension after rapid sequence intubation. *Am J Emerg Med* 26:845–851.

Martyn JA, Richtsfeld M (2006) Succinylcholine-induced hyperkalemia in acquired pathologic states: etiologic factors and molecular mechanisms. *Anesthesiology* 104:158–169.

Case 188

Ghanem T, Rasamny JK, Park SS (2005) Rethinking auricular trauma. *Laryngoscope* 115:1251–1255.

Giles WC, Iverson KC, King JD *et al.* (2007) Incision and drainage followed by mattress suture repair of auricular hematoma. *Laryngoscope* 117:2097–2099.

Case 189

Aslam AF, Aslam AK, Vasavada BC *et al.* (2006) Hypothermia: evaluation, electrocardiographic manifestations, and management. *Am J Med* 119:297–301.

Vassallo SU, Delaney KA, Hoffman RS *et al.* (1999) A prospective evaluation of the electrocardiographic manifestations of hypothermia. *Acad Emerg Med* 6:1121–1126.

Case 190

Knobloch K, Wagner S, Haasper C *et al.* (2008) Sternal fractures are frequent among polytraumatised patients following high deceleration velocities in a severe vehicle crash. *Injury* 39:36–43.

Recinos G, Inaba K, Dubose J *et al.* (2009) Epidemiology of sternal fractures. *Am Surg* 75:401–404.

Case 191

Frolkis JP, Pothier CE, Blackstone E H *et al.* (2003) Frequent ventricular ectopy after exercise as a predictor of death. *N Engl J Med* 348:781–790.

Lerma C, Lee CF, Glass L *et al.* (2007) The rule of bigeminy revisited: analysis in sudden cardiac death syndrome. *J Electrocardiol* 40:78–88.

Case 192

Robinett DA, Shelton B, Dyer KS (2010) Special consideration in hazardous materials burns. *J Emerg Med* 39:544–553.

Stratta RJ , Saffle JR, Kravitz M *et al.* (1983) Management of tar and asphalt injuries. *Am J Surg* 146:766–769.

Case 193

Kinzer S, Pfeiffer J, Becker S *et al.* (2009) Severe deep neck space infections and mediastinitis of odontogenic origin: clinical relevance and implications for diagnosis and treatment. *Acta Otolaryngol* 129:62–70.

Marioni G, Rinaldi R, Staffieri C *et al.* (2008) Deep neck infection with dental origin: analysis of 85 consecutive cases (2000–2006). *Acta Otolaryngol* 128:201–206.

Case 194

Patel RV, DeLong W Jr, Vresilovic EJ (2004) Evaluation and treatment of spinal injuries in the patient with polytrauma. *Clin Orthop Rel Res* 422:43–54.

Sciubba DM, Petteys RJ(2009) Evaluation of blunt cervical spine injury. *South Med J* **102**:823–828.

Case 195
Lubner M, Menias C, Rucker C *et al.* (2007) Blood in the belly: CT findings of hemoperitoneum. *Radiographics* **27**:109–125.
Shanley CJ, Weinberger JB (2008) Acute abdominal vascular emergencies. *Med Clin North Am* **92**:627–647.

Case 196
Abecasis J, Monge J, Alberca D *et al.* (2008) Electrocardiographic presentation of massive and submassive pulmonary embolism. *Rev Port Cardiol* **27**:591–610.
Ullman E, Brady WJ, Perron AD *et al.* (2001) Electrocardiographic manifestations of pulmonary embolism. *Am J Emerg Med* **19**:514–519.

Case 197
Golledge J, Eagle KA (2008) Acute aortic dissection. *Lancet* **372**:55–66.
Kamalakannan D, Rosman HS, Eagle KA (2007) Acute aortic dissection. *Crit Care Clin* **23**:779–800.

Case 198
Karger S, Führer D (2008) Thyroid storm: thyrotoxic crisis: an update. *Dtsch Med Wochenschr* **133**:479–484.
Nayak B, Burman K (2006) Thyrotoxicosis and thyroid storm. *Endocrinol Metab Clin North Am* **35**:663–686.

Case 199
Patel RV, Weinberg JM (2008) Psoriasis in the patient with human immunodeficiency virus, part 1: review of pathogenesis. *Cutis* **82**:117–122.
Patel RV, Weinberg JM (2008) Psoriasis in the patient with human immunodeficiency virus, part 2: review of treatment. *Cutis* **82**:202–210.

Case 200
Bedi DG, Gombos DS, Ng CS *et al.* (2006) Sonography of the eye. *Am J Roentgenol* **187**:1061–1072.
D'Amico DJ (2008) Clinical practice: primary retinal detachment. *N Engl J Med* **359**:2346–2354.

Case 201
Garcia HH, Del Brutto OH, Nash TE *et al.* (2005) New concepts in the diagnosis and management of neurocysticercosis (*Taenia solium*). *Am J Trop Med Hyg* **72**:3–9.
Ramírez-Zamora A, Alarcón T (2010) Management of neurocysticercosis. *Neurol Res* **32**:229–237.

Case 202
Udekwu P, Kromhout-Schiro S, Vaslef S *et al.* (2004) Glasgow Coma Scale score, mortality, and functional outcome in head-injured patients. *J Trauma* **56**:1084–1089.
Zuercher M, Ummenhofer W, Baltussen A *et al.* (2009) The use of Glasgow Coma Scale in injury assessment: a critical review. *Brain Inj* **23**:371–384.

Case 203
Sakalihasan N, Limet R, Defawe O D (2005) Abdominal aortic aneurysm. *Lancet* **365**:1577–1589.
Visser JJ, van Sambeek MR, Hamza TH *et al.* (2007) Ruptured abdominal aortic aneurysms: endovascular repair versus open surgery: systematic review. *Radiology* **245**:122–129.

Case 204
Anglen JO, Archdeacon MT, Cannada LK *et al.* (2008) Avoiding complications in the treatment of humeral fractures. *J Bone Joint Surg Am Vol* **90**:1580–1589.
Shao YC, Harwood P, Grotz MR *et al.* (2005) Radial nerve palsy associated with fractures of the shaft of the humerus: a systematic review. *J Bone Joint Surg Br* **87**:1647–1652.

Further reading

Case 205

Collignon NJ (2005) Emergencies in glaucoma: a review. *Bull Belg Ophthalmol Soc* **296**:71–81.

Lam DS, Tham CC, Lai JS *et al.* (2007) Current approaches to the management of acute primary angle closure. *Curr Opin Ophthalmol* **18**:146–151.

Case 206

Kowalsky MS, Levine WN (2008) Traumatic posterior glenohumeral dislocation: classification, pathoanatomy, diagnosis, and treatment. *Orthop Clin North Am* **39**:519–533.

Robinson CM, Aderinto J (2005) Posterior shoulder dislocations and fracture-dislocations. *J Bone Joint Surg Am Vol* **87**:639–650.

Case 207

Benito B, Brugada R, Brugada J *et al.* (2008) Brugada syndrome. *Prog Cardiovasc Dis* **51**:1–22.

Boussy T, Sarkozy A, Chierchia GB *et al.* (2007) The Brugada syndrome: facts and controversies. *Herz* **32**:192–200.

Case 208

Korownyk C, Allan GM (2007) Evidence-based approach to abscess management. *Can Fam Physician* **53**:1680–1684.

Rogers RL, Perkins J (2006) Skin and soft tissue infections. *Prim Care* **33**:697–710.

Case 209

Dhar S, Lidhoo P, Koul D *et al.* (2009) Current concepts and management strategies in atrial flutter. *South Med J* **102**:917–922.

Khan IA, Nair CK, Singh N *et al.* (2004) Acute ventricular rate control in atrial fibrillation and atrial flutter. *Int J Cardiol* **97**:7–13.

Case 210

Ahmad F, Turner SA, Torrie P *et al.* (2008) Iatrogenic femoral artery pseudoaneurysms: a review of current methods of diagnosis and treatment. *Clin Radiol* **63**:1310–1316.

Bechara C, Huynh TT, Lin PH (2007) Management of lower extremity arterial injuries. *J Cardiovasc Surg* **48**:567–579.

Case 211

Robinson-Bostom L, DiGiovanna JJ (2000) Cutaneous manifestations of end-stage renal disease. *J Am Acad Dermatol* **43**:975–986.

Udayakumar P, Balasubramanian S, Ramalingam KS *et al.* (2006) Cutaneous manifestations in patients with chronic renal failure on hemodialysis. *Indian J Dermatol Venereol Leprol* **72**:119–125.

Case 212

Dykewicz MS, Hamilos DL (2010) Rhinitis and sinusitis. *J Allergy Clin Immunol* **125**(Suppl 2):S103–115.

Small CB, Bachert C, Lund VJ *et al.* (2007) Judicious antibiotic use and intranasal corticosteroids in acute rhinosinusitis. *Am J Med* **120**:289–294.

Case 213

Fangman JJ, Scadden DT (2005) Anemia in HIV-infected adults: epidemiology, pathogenesis, and clinical management. *Curr Hematol Rep* **4**:95–102.

McEwen MP, Bull GP, Reynolds KJ (2009) Vessel calibre and haemoglobin effects on pulse oximetry. *Physiol Meas* **30**:869–883.

Case 214

Bullock MR, Chesnut R, Ghajar J *et al.* (2006) Surgical management of acute epidural hematomas. *Neurosurgery* **58**(3Suppl):S7–15.

Radulovic D, Janosevic V, Djurovic B *et al.* (2006) Traumatic delayed epidural hematoma. *Zentralbl Neurochir* **67**:76–80.

Case 215

Hou W, Sanyal AJ (2009) Ascites: diagnosis and management. *Med Clin North Am* **93**:801–817.

Kuiper JJ, de Man RA, van Buuren HR (2007) Review article: management of ascites and associated complications in patients with cirrhosis. *Alim Pharmacol Therap* **26(Suppl 2)**:183–193.

Case 216

Caceres M, Braud RL, Maekawa R *et al.* (2009) Secondary pneumomediastinum: a retrospective comparative analysis. *Lung* **187**:341–346.

Dissanaike S, Shalhub S, Jurkovich GJ (2008) The evaluation of pneumomediastinum in blunt trauma patients. *J Trauma* **65**:1340–1345.

Case 217

Cáceres-Lóriga FM, Pérez-López H, Morlans-Hernández K *et al.* (2006) Thrombolysis as first choice therapy in prosthetic heart valve thrombosis: a study of 68 patients. *J Thromb Thrombol* **21**:185–190.

Cáceres-Lóriga FM, Pérez-López H, Santos-Gracia J *et al.* (2006) Prosthetic heart valve thrombosis: pathogenesis, diagnosis and management. *Int J Cardiol* **110**:1–6.

Case 218

Moeller JL (2003) Pelvic and hip apophyseal avulsion injuries in young athletes. *Curr Sports Med Rep* **2**:110–115.

Sanders TG, Zlatkin MB (2008) Avulsion injuries of the pelvis. *Semin Musculoskelet Radiol* **12**:42–53.

Case 219

Grossman NB (2004) Blunt trauma in pregnancy. *Am Fam Physician* **70**:1303–1310.

Petrone P, Asensio JA (2006) Trauma in pregnancy: assessment and treatment. *Scand J Surg* **95**:4–10.

Case 220

Sherrid MV (2006) Pathophysiology and treatment of hypertrophic cardiomyopathy. *Prog Cardiovasc Dis* **49**:123–151.

Soor GS, Luk A, Ahn E *et al.* (2009) Hypertrophic cardiomyopathy: current understanding and treatment objectives. *J Clin Pathol* **62**:226–235.

Case 221

Gammons MG, Jackson E (2001) Fishhook removal. *Am Fam Physician* **63**:2231–2236.

Ma HP, Lin AC (2005) A simple method for removal of fish hooks in the emergency department. *Br J Sports Med* **39**:116–117.

Case 222

McGillicuddy D, Rosen P (2007) Diagnostic dilemmas and current controversies in blunt chest trauma. *Emerg Med Clin North Am* **25**:695–711.

Tekeli A, Akgun S (2004) Blunt chest trauma and tube thoracostomy. *Ann Thorac Surg* **77**:754–755.

Case 223

Iwatsuki K, Yamasaki O, Morizane S *et al.* (2006) Staphylococcal cutaneous infections: invasion, evasion and aggression. *J Dermatol Sci* **42**:203–214.

Ong YK, Chee G (2005) Infections of the external ear. *Ann Acad Med Singapore* **34**:330–334.

Case 224

Tay JC, Chee YC (1998) Ergotism and vascular insufficiency: a case report and review of literature. *Ann Acad Med Singapore* **27**:285–288.

Zavaleta EG, Fernandez BB, Grove M K *et al.* (2001) St. Anthony's fire (ergotamine induced leg ischemia): a case report and review of the literature. *Angiology* **52**:349–356.

Further reading

Case 225
Iakobishvili Z, Hasdai D (2007)
Cardiogenic shock: treatment. *Med Clin North Am* **91**:713–727.
Topalian S, Ginsberg F, Parrillo JE (2008)
Cardiogenic shock. *Crit Care Med* **36**(1 Suppl):S66–74.

Case 226
Mathura KC, Thapa N, Rauniyar A *et al.*
(2005) Injection drug use and tricuspid valve endocarditis. *Kathmandu Univ Med J* **3**:84–86.
Yung D, Kottachchi D, Neupane B *et al.*
(2007) Antimicrobials for right-sided endocarditis in intravenous drug users: a systematic review. *J Antimicrob Chemother* **60**:921–928.

Case 227
Evans KJ, Greenberg A (2005)
Hyperkalemia: a review. *J Intensive Care Med* **20**:272–290.
Weisberg LS (2008) Management of severe hyperkalemia. *Crit Care Med* **36**:3246–3251.

Case 228
Harrop JS, Sharan A, Ratliff J (2006)
Central cord injury: pathophysiology, management, and outcomes. *Spine J* **6**(6 Suppl):198S–206S.
Pollard ME, Apple DF (2003) Factors associated with improved neurologic outcomes in patients with incomplete tetraplegia. *Spine* **28**:33–39.

Case 229
Lambrecht RW, Thapar M, Bonkovsky HL (2007) Genetic aspects of porphyria cutanea tarda. *Semin Liver Dis* **27**:99–108.
Sassa S (2006) Modern diagnosis and management of the porphyrias. *Br J Haematol* **135**:281–292.

Case 230
Brown DJ, Jaffe JE, Henson JK (2007)
Advanced laceration management. *Emerg Med Clin North Am* **25**:83–99.
Wilson JL, Kocurek K, Doty BJ (2000) A systematic approach to laceration repair: tricks to ensure the desired cosmetic result. *Postgrad Med* **107**:77–83, 87–88.

Case 231
Barnhart KT (2009) Clinical practice: ectopic pregnancy. *N Engl J Med* **361**:379–387.
Bhatt S, Ghazale H, Dogra VS (2007)
Sonographic evaluation of ectopic pregnancy. *Radiol Clin North Am* **45**:549–560.

Case 232
Rosner MH, Brady WJ Jr, Kefer MP *et al.*
(1999) Electrocardiography in the patient with the Wolff-Parkinson-White syndrome: diagnostic and initial therapeutic issues. *Am J Emerg Med* **17**:705–714.
Tischenko A, Fox DJ, Yee R *et al.* (2008)
When should we recommend catheter ablation for patients with the Wolff-Parkinson-White syndrome? *Curr Opin Cardiol* **23**:32–37.

Case 233
Aoyama H, Tanaka M, Hara M *et al.*
(1999) Nummular eczema: an addition of senile xerosis and unique cutaneous reactivities to environmental aeroallergens. *Dermatology* **199**:135–139.
Järvikallio A, Harvima IT, Naukkarinen A (2003) Mast cells, nerves and neuropeptides in atopic dermatitis and nummular eczema. *Arch Dermatol Res* **295**:2–7.

Case 234

Caldicott DG, Pearce A, Price R *et al.* (2004) Not just another 'head lac'...low-velocity, penetrating intra-cranial injuries: a case report and review of the literature. *Injury* **35**:1044–1054.

Martin S, Raup GH, Cravens G *et al.* (2009) Management of embedded foreign body: penetrating stab wound to the head. *J Trauma Nurs* **16**:82–86.

Case 235

Díaz-Manera J, Rojas-García R, Illa I (2009) Treatment strategies for myasthenia gravis. *Expert Opin Pharmacother* **10**:1329–1342.

Juel VC, Massey JM (2007) Myasthenia gravis. *Orphanet J Rare Dis* **2**:44.

Case 236

Das D, Ali B (2003) Towards evidence based emergency medicine: best BETs from the Manchester Royal Infirmary: conservative management of asymptomatic cocaine body packers. *Emerg Med J* **20**:172–174.

de Prost N, Lefebvre A, Questel F *et al.* (2005) Prognosis of cocaine body-packers. *Intensive Care Med* **31**:955–958.

Case 237

Requena L, Sánchez Yus E (2007) Erythema nodosum. *Semin Cutan Med Surg* **26**:114–125.

Requena L, Yus ES (2008) Erythema nodosum. *Dermatol Clin* **26**:425–438.

Case 238

Chiquet C, Zech JC, Denis P *et al.* (1999) Intraocular foreign bodies: factors influencing final visual outcome. *Acta Ophthalmol Scand* **77**:321–325.

Ehlers JP, Kunimoto DY, Ittoop S *et al.* (2008) Metallic intraocular foreign bodies: characteristics, interventions, and prognostic factors for visual outcome and globe survival. *Am J Ophthalmol* **146**:427–433.

Case 239

Boden WE, Gupta V (2009) Acute coronary syndromes: selective vs early invasive strategies. *Clin Cardiol* **32**:621–626.

Thomas D, Giugliano RP (2010) Day 1 care in patients with non-ST-segment elevation myocardial infarction. *Cardiovasc Revasc Med* **11**:41–51.

Case 240

Khan LA, Bradnock TJ, Scott C *et al.* (2009) Fractures of the clavicle. *J Bone Joint Surg Am Vol* **91**:447–460.

Kim W, McKee MD (2008) Management of acute clavicle fractures. *Orthop Clin North Am* **39**:491–505.

Case 241

Mueller JB, McStay CM (2008) Ocular infection and inflammation. *Emerg Med Clin North Am* **26**:57–72.

Paranjpe DR, Foulks GN (2003) Therapy for meibomian gland disease. *Ophthalmol Clin North Am* **16**:37–42.

Case 242

Martró E, Esteve A, Schulz TF *et al.* (2007) Risk factors for human Herpesvirus 8 infection and AIDS-associated Kaposi's sarcoma among men who have sex with men in a European multicentre study. *Int J Cancer* **120**:1129–1135.

Stebbing J, Sanitt A, Nelson M *et al.* (2006) A prognostic index for AIDS-associated Kaposi's sarcoma in the era of highly active antiretroviral therapy. *Lancet* **367**:1495–1502.

Case 243

Budoff JE (2008) Treatment of acute lunate and perilunate dislocations. *J Hand Surg* **33**:1424–1432.

Perron AD, Brady WJ, Keats TE *et al.* (2001) Orthopedic pitfalls in the ED: lunate and perilunate injuries. *Am J Emerg Med* **19**:157–162.

Further reading

Case 244

Watkinson AF, Yeow TN, Fraser C (2008) Endovascular stenting to treat obstruction of the superior vena cava. *BMJ* **336**:1434–1437.

Wilson LD, Detterbeck FC, Yahalom J (2007) Clinical practice: superior vena cava syndrome with malignant causes. *N Engl J Med* **356**:1862–1869.

Case 245

Rinkenberger RL, Polumbo RA, Bolton MR *et al.* (1978) Mechanism of electrical alternans in patients with pericardial effusion. *Cathet Cardiovasc Diagn* **4**:63–70.

Spencker S, Müller D, Mochmann HC (2008) Pericardial effusion and electrical alternans. *Resuscitation* **76**:163–164.

Case 246

Baron RL, Tublin ME, Peterson MS (2002) Imaging the spectrum of biliary tract disease. *Radiol Clin North Am* **40**:1325–1354.

Keus F, Broeders IA, van Laarhoven CJ (2006) Gallstone disease: surgical aspects of symptomatic cholecystolithiasis and acute cholecystitis. *Best Pract Res Clin Gastroenterol* **20**:1031–1051.

Case 247

Hobgood ER, Khan SO, Field LD (2008) Acute dislocations of the adult elbow. *Hand Clin* **24**:1–7.

Kuhn MA, Ross G (2008) Acute elbow dislocations. *Orthop Clin North Am* **39**:155–161.

Case 248

Makarovsky I, Markel G, Dushnitsky T *et al.* (2008) Hydrogen fluoride: the protoplasmic poison. *Isr Med Assoc J* **10**:381–385.

Salzman M, O'Malley RN (2007) Updates on the evaluation and management of caustic exposures. *Emerg Med Clin North Am* **25**:459–476.

Case 249

Dix FP, Khan Y, Al-Khaffaf H (2006) The brachial artery-basilic vein arterio-venous fistula in vascular access for haemodialysis: a review paper. *Eur J Vasc Endovasc Surg* **31**:70–79.

Hossny A (2003) Brachiobasilic arteriovenous fistula: different surgical techniques and their effects on fistula patency and dialysis-related complications. *J Vasc Surg* **37**:821–826.

Case 250

Manchanda V, Gupta S, Bhalla P (2006) Meningococcal disease: history, epidemiology, pathogenesis, clinical manifestations, diagnosis, antimicrobial susceptibility and prevention. *Indian J Med Microbiol* **24**:7–19.

Stephens DS (2007) Conquering the meningococcus. *FEMS Microbiol Rev* **31**:3–14.

Case 251

Ramaraj R (2010) Peripartum cardiomyopathy. *Minerva Ginecol* **62**:129–136.

Yamac H, Bultmann I, Sliwa K *et al.* (2010) Prolactin: a new therapeutic target in peripartum cardiomyopathy. *Heart* **96**:1352–1357.

Index

Index

Index